S K
R U L E S

ADVANCE PRAISE FOR THE BOOK

'This gem of a book is a comprehensive compilation that will take you from the essentials of self-preservation to the most complex layered technology services available, and everything in between'—Amitabh Bachchan, actor

'Dearest Jaishree, you continue to make me proud with your many accomplishments and the admiration of your colleagues. You have always been my favourite student'—Stephen Mandy, renowned cosmetic dermatologist, Miami

'Your skin at times can be your arch-nemesis, working against you and becoming something you constantly need to be aware of and wary of. When someone like Jaishree enters your life, you feel like you have won the skin battle! She makes the cure painless and immediately effective—it's an "ageless" bond and your skin's BFF for life'—Karan Johar, director

'As the largest organ of the body, the skin is literally a window into the type of lifestyle you are living. Healthy skin not only makes you feel more youthful but also signals your vibrancy to others. Dr Jaishree Sharad is a well-respected colleague and internationally recognized skin expert. I have personally learnt so much from her and it is wonderful that her tricks are now in print for everyone to keep looking their best'—Kavita Mariwala, renowned cosmetic dermatologist, New York

'Dr Jaishree Sharad sums up the take-home points on the daily skincare routine, making it easy and very doable. Her book sheds light on the esoteric and makes taking care of your largest organ accessible to all. A must-read'—Hassan Galadari, renowned cosmetic dermatologist, Dubai

'You are an international derm diva!'—Heidi Waldorf, renowned cosmetic dermatologist, New York

'Dear Jaishree, I am very happy to witness your success as a teacher. There is no more happiness for an old teacher like me than seeing my trainee carry on my mission. Congratulations on your success, my daughter from India'—Dr Niwat Polnikorn, renowned cosmetic dermatologist, Bangkok

'I am an old man but I look more presentable and younger than I did twenty years ago! The complete credit goes to none other than my darling Dr Jaishree Sharad! She believes in care and cure and not commercial viability, and that makes her one in a million!

बरसते रहो सावन सरीखे खेत में
महकते रहो चंदन सरीखे देश में
लोग तो मिट्टी से सोना ही निकालें
और तुम मोती उगाओ रेत में
—Annu Kapoor, actor

'Jaishree is so knowledgeable about the latest developments in skincare that makes it easier for you to look younger and fresher. There is no one better than her to write a book on skincare because we want our outer beauty to match the inner beauty'—Farah Khan, director

'I get dark circles when I don't sleep . . . I get sunburnt and my skin peels when I spend the day on the beach . . . I break out into pimples and acne when I'm stressed . . . But as a film star, I've gotta always look like I've walked out of a magazine cover! That's when I realized great skin doesn't happen by chance, it happens by appointment . . . Dr Jaishree is my one-stop shop. Forget the camera, she's the reason I look into the mirror!'—Ranbir Kapoor, actor

'I have been going to Dr Jaishree for several years and there is no one I trust more to take care of my skin. She always has apt advice and a fantastic bedside manner that makes the treatment painless and stress-free. She does not overprescribe and makes sure you take care of your health through food and fluids. My husband tells me that I see her more often than my best friend, but I always go to her for the best and the right advice'—Sonam Kapoor, actor

'As an actor, I am always on the move, working with few hours of sleep and a schedule which is not skin-friendly. Jaishree is my instant cure for any skin problem. Whether I get any scar or pimple or mark, she is "Dr Solve It" for me'—Varun Dhawan, actor

'One thing I have noticed is that the oxygen facials at Dr J's Skinfiniti work well when you drink a lot of water, get good sleep and take vitamin C. Ghee in my coffee has also helped in making my skin look naturally moisturized'—Jacqueline Fernandez, actor

'I had pimples and scars on my face all my life and I struggled with them. Then I met Dr J and she did her magic. Now I smile and have dimples instead of pimples. I also have the pleasure of knowing this beautiful being personally'—Amit Sadh, actor

'Jaishree is undoubtedly one of the best in the business. She is not of those who constantly highlight the flaws in our features and lure us into trying new treatments. She will do only what is necessary and knows when to stop, so I feel completely safe in her hands. I have a very sensitive skin, so I do not like doing too much to it, but her mesotherapy treatment once a month is a must for me. Being good at work is great, but for me being a good human always comes first—and Jaishree is one of the nicest, most genuine, caring and positive souls I have come across, and I love her even more for that. I am so proud of all her achievements'—Shamita Shetty, actor

'I've been visiting Dr J's clinic for several years now . . . and there's no one else I trust with my skin. She doesn't believe in extreme and radical treatments. She is so quick and accurate with her diagnosis. I have sensitive skin and face various skin issues. I make it a point to keep her in the loop and see her twice a month. With very little downtime and the lack of appropriate treatments, as well as spot-on advice, she is the best. Instead of self-medicating and trying to find solutions on the Internet, try and make an appointment with your dermatologist. Otherwise you could permanently damage your skin. Sometimes a healthy diet and lifestyle aren't enough. You need a qualified professional to look at your skin and an equally skilful pair of hands to do your skin treatments'—Harshvardhan Kapoor, actor

'I have always taken my skin for granted and treated it like an outward part of my body. Jaishree taught me the importance of loving my skin and nourishing it—that less is always more. She is my go-to person in times of panic because she can cure with immediate effect and calm my nerves too'—Athiya Shetty, actor

'Dr J has been my skin saviour. Before every shoot, I consult her on the best possible skin routine to follow depending on the weather conditions I am shooting in. I remember calling her after I got badly sunburnt during a particular schedule and was in tears and she sorted me out immediately. I have sensitive skin and it reacts to changes in weather and my diet a lot. Thanks to her, my skincare routine has become really easy!'—Huma Qureshi, actor

'I'm yet to come across a more passionate and well-informed doctor. The medical profession is perhaps one of a kind where the process of learning never stops. That's where I think Dr Jaishree Sharad scores the most. I know her now since 2009, and as we have evolved in age, she has evolved in methods and techniques'—Nikhil Dwivedi, actor and producer

'I've been Dr J's patient since 2015. I used to suffer from pimples and dull skin. Today my skin glows and is pimple-free thanks to Jaishree and her easy procedures. The peels she has done on my skin have worked wonders. More importantly, the stem cell PRP hair treatment has really helped me battle my hair loss issues'—Amyra Dastur, actor

'As a guy in his early twenties, I never really thought of going to a dermatologist. But after my first session with Dr Jaishree, I realized how much I could and should take care of my skin. From the word go she made me comfortable and confident in my own skin. The "Skinfiniti Signature clean-up" is my personal favourite. I always leave the clinic feeling revitalized and rejuvenated'—Aadar Jain, actor

'I make sure that I drink lots of water and eat plenty of fruits because it keeps my skin fresh and hydrated. Applying aloe vera on my skin also works like magic! Sleep is important too but when sometimes work does not give you the sleep your body requires, break-outs or skin reactions do happen. But the good thing is that Jaishree will always be available and ready to help'—Elli Avram, actor

'You're the best doc, and thank you helping me out with my skin'— Karan Kapadia, actor

'For someone who backpacks often and is not diligent with skincare or beautification, it was a blessing to meet Dr Jaishree. She simplified things and helped me understand the essence of skincare through the most essential and non-fussy of regimens. I deeply admire her positive energy and warmth. She is a slice of home'—Sobhita Dhulipala, actor

'It has been more than ten years and Jaishree is the only dermatologist I trust with any skin issue—not only me but my family and friends too. Today, she is a world-renowned doctor and that is a huge achievement'—Ehsaan Noorani, music composer

'Healthy and glowing skin is very important for a person's confidence. I try to be as natural as I can and always vouch for home remedies like besan or yogurt packs once in a while. I believe in cleansing my skin well and getting rid of all the make-up before sleep and letting it breathe overnight. Also, drinking water to keep your skin hydrated is really important. Skin tips from Dr J and basic peels and face packs at Skinfiniti have also changed the way my skin looks and feels'—Priya Banerjee, actor

'Love J! She is the best'—Shekhar Ravjiani, musician

'I always had a decent skin—clear with occasional break-outs. But when I started with my first film, my face suddenly broke out. Every doctor I visited gave me hundreds of expensive products—my skin only got worse. It was then that I met Dr Jaishree. She took time to understand what my skin was like before I started acting and immediately realized that the new make-up was the culprit. It was so simple yet no one else before had realized it. I switched make-up brands, stopped using all the unnecessary products and saw an immediate improvement. She gave me a simple routine (cleanser and moisturizer) and with regular clean-ups at her clinic, my skin has been better! I love her because she never pushes products on you and only addresses your concern in simple and effective ways. The fact that she is one of the sweetest people is also a plus!'—Kalyani Priyadarshan, actor

'What can I say about Jaishree Sharad? As a person she is one of the loveliest people I know. She is kind and gentle. She has a lovely smile. She's always happy and full of life. Even when she is not, she appears to be. As a doctor she is someone whom I can trust wholeheartedly. There are lots of times when I want to do treatments but she doesn't let me because she says I don't need it. I think that is one of her best qualities—that she doesn't force you to do anything. She looks at your face, evaluates it and then decides what kind of treatment is needed. She doesn't sell you anything. I can tell you that my face has never looked better and it's all thanks to her. Thank you, doctor. I love you'—Yasmin Karachiwala, celebrity fitness expert

'She is the best doctor in the world! I wouldn't go to anyone else. Fantastic dermatologist, an amazing person and my best friend' —Namrata Dutt Kumar, social worker

'Jaishree is my best friend, guide and go-to person for everything. She is one person I can truly trust with closed eyes. She is also a fantastic doctor. Thank you, Jaishree, for always putting up with me. I am so proud of you'—Riddhima Kapoor, designer

'J is not only my go-to person when I need skin advice, she is a dear friend too. I wish her all the best for *Skin Rules*'—Poorna Patel

'When you feel good, you look good. That happens when you meet Dr Jaishree. She is such a warm and positive person, her smile and kindness makes you feel good even before you start the treatment. I have the confidence that she will guide me to choose the right treatments for my skin'—Iulia Vantur, singer

'I leave my skincare routine to Dr Jaishree. Whether it is hydration, diet or oxygen facials, Jaishree knows best. As a doctor, she has no shortcuts to a good and healthy life'—Jitesh Pillai, editor

'JS is not just a skin doctor. She is also a skin and mind healer. She heals her patients not just physically but by even instilling self-confidence and happiness in her clients. She is a real-life heroine—a beautiful, giving, caring, compassionate, intelligent and extremely hard-working being whose aura is what I seek when I feel under the weather'—Shalini Sharma

'My experience with Dr Jaishree has been a kind of revolution for my skin! It completely changed my perception and understanding of skincare! When I met her for the first time, I had plenty of skin issues being a teenager. After going through several vigorous skincare routines as prescribed by different dermatologists, her guidance was refreshing! She gave me a very simple, basic routine to follow without any heavy medication or treatments and it worked magically! I have a sensitive skin . . . My profession involves travelling to different places, late-night shoots, being under the light for hours and that leads to frequent skin emergencies. Whenever I call her with a skin crisis (break-outs and such), she just tells me, "Calm down, Palak, I'll sort it out." Her expertise, warmth and concern make me feel relieved about any skin problem I may have. My skin is in its best form today and it's only because of her! My skin saviour!'—Palak Muchhal, singer

'Your expertise and knowledge are always up to the mark and the results prove it each time! I've known you for years now and have always had a great experience! And not to forget, your staff is as sweet and nice as you are'—Gaurie Pandit Dwivedi

'Expert hands with a human touch! She's as personal as she is professional. Dr Jaishree is one of the most passionate, honest and sincere doctors I have come across. I completely trust her with all my worries and concerns and she takes care of them perfectly'—Prithvi Hatte, actor

'I took my husband to Dr Jaishree Sharad and now he looks younger than me. Dr J has magical hands! She is truly the best!'—Anupama Kapoor

SKIN
RULES

Your 6-week plan to radiant skin

DR JAISHREE SHARAD

EBURY
PRESS

An imprint of Penguin Random House

EBURY PRESS

USA | Canada | UK | Ireland | Australia
New Zealand | India | South Africa | China

Ebury Press is part of the Penguin Random House group of companies
whose addresses can be found at global.penguinrandomhouse.com

Published by Penguin Random House India Pvt. Ltd
7th Floor, Infinity Tower C, DLF Cyber City,
Gurgaon 122 002, Haryana, India

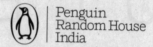

First published in Ebury Press by Penguin Random House India 2018

Illustrations by Pooja Mertia

ISBN 9780143444725

Typeset in Sabon by Manipal Digital Systems, Manipal
Printed at Thomson Press India Ltd, New Delhi

www.penguin.co.in

To my daddy—an engineer par excellence, an amazing artist, a fabulous teacher, a genius in every way. He was the strong, silent pillar behind every milestone in my life. I sat in his room and wrote this book. I am sure he was sitting next to me and giving me all the ideas. Dear Daddy, I am sorry I read your diary without your permission. You said I did you proud. I hope this book will do you more proud even up there in heaven.

I miss you.

Contents

Contents

Introduction

I completed my MBBS in 1995 and went on to do my post-graduation in dermatology. Apart from dealing with problems related to skin, I was also trained in dermatologic surgery, which involved chemical peels, lasers, vitiligo surgery, acne scar reduction and so on.

I was the first dermatologic surgeon to start practice in Navi Mumbai, in January 2000. At that time, my husband was a junior surgeon in one of the reputed hospitals of Navi Mumbai. I wanted to do a fellowship in cosmetic dermatology somewhere in the US because I needed to fine-tune my Botox and filler injection skills. But that would involve heavy costs, which we couldn't afford. So I started to visit five different polyclinics and one hospital as a consultant dermatologist, my working hours being from 10 a.m. to 10 p.m.

In June 2004, I got the opportunity to do a fellowship in cosmetic dermatology in Bangkok. By now I had saved up a little money to sustain my added expenses in a different country. It was my first-ever international trip, at the age of thirty. That is where my journey as a cosmetic dermatologist began. Later I also underwent training in cosmetic dermatology in Miami, North Carolina and Los Angeles.

June 2006 saw the birth of Skinfiniti, one in Vashi and one in Bandra, and there has been no looking back since. Through my journey, I realized how people lacked knowledge about skin. It used to bother me when I saw people giving importance to all the organs of the body except the skin. Not only that, most rashes, pimples, pigmentation are treated with home remedies which further ruin the skin.

So when Milee Ashwarya, the publisher of Random House India, asked me to write a book, I decided to take the plunge. My first book, *Skin Talks*, was published in 2014. This book has a detailed description of the anatomy of skin, nagging skin problems, product ingredients, skin in different climates, etc. Though the book has been a bestseller, a few of my younger patients said it was too elaborate and they'd rather come to me and take a prescription. In 2017 when Milee coaxed me into writing another book, I decided to adapt to the changing world and cater to the generation which functions at a fast pace.

They say, when in Rome, do as the Romans do. So I decided to write a more simple, illustrative book which a teenager could enjoy as much as an eighty-year-old could.

My editor Gurveen came up with the brilliant idea of six weeks to radiant skin. 'It is impossible! One would need at least three months,' I told Gurveen. We were playing tug of war with no outcome. Around the same time, a patient—let's call her Mickey—came to my clinic. And guess what, she wanted flawless skin in six weeks! Perhaps it was God's way of telling me to take up Gurveen's challenge.

'Dr J, I want my skin to be radiant and glowing. Not just six weeks from now, but for ever after. I can't be sitting with make-up at home, especially when my mother-in-law-to-be is the most stylish lady I have seen. So please do some magic,' Mickey said. Obviously, she had come to me with a lot of hope and there was no way I could let her down. I examined her skin with my magnifying glass, and then my skin analyser. (A skin analyser comes with a powerful camera and functions which help to peep into the deeper layers of the skin and analyse skin irregularities, levels of pigmentation, as well as fungal and bacterial infections of the skin.)

Mickey's skin was dull and blotchy. She had a few whiteheads on her forehead and blackheads on her nose. Her eyes looked tired and she had just about started to develop dark circles.

We had an elaborate chat about her eating and drinking habits, her lifestyle, work and stress levels and, of course, her skincare regime. Mickey was a super-busy entrepreneur. She worked late nights, slept very little, partied hard, smoked occasionally, ate whatever she could lay hands on (though she claimed she ate healthy), barely exercised because she did not have the time. And skincare was alien to her.

To top it all, she was stressed and running around in the sun for her many last-minute wedding preparations.

I took a deep breath as I spoke to her, as if convincing myself that I could meet this flawless-skin challenge only if she cooperated. I had to make sure that by the end of six weeks, Mickey had an even skin tone, i.e. her skin had a uniform colour. Her skin texture had to be smooth and supple. Her skin had to be devoid of blemishes or pimples. She had to have no dark circles, fine lines or open pores. And of course she had to look like a million bucks. A few skin creams wouldn't do the trick, nor would a laser work like a magic wand. I made her promise she would follow my instructions to a T and carefully chalked out a plan for her.

That night, I went home and wrote an email to Gurveen—*Six weeks to radiant skin it is!*

Skin Rules, we called it, and here it is in your hands. Mickey is representative of every patient of mine who yearns for clear skin. She is the face of every individual, male or female, who wants to look good but is tired of searching for answers on the Internet or in beauty shops. In an era where cosmetic and pharmaceutical companies make billions of dollars on skincare products, the Internet doesn't have honest or relevant answers all the time. Packaging, marketing and advertisements have a strong influence on sales of any skincare product or even skin treatment.

Mickey is every individual who does not want to get deceived but wants genuine guidance. I know of a lot of boys who use their sisters' creams and a lot of men who empty their wives' closets because they are uncomfortable buying skincare products in the store. That skincare is vanity and only for women is but a false belief. Mickey is every guy's voice too because glowing skin is not a 'female' thing.

Finally, I am not a writer. I am just another dermatologist who wants to spread awareness about skin and skincare. I must have edited each sentence five times just to make you understand the context better. I have pondered over all the common skin issues my patients face in their day-to-day lives. And I have tried to find some simple solutions and put them in my weekly programme.

Though an ideal pathway to glowing skin, especially if there are problems such as acne or pigmentation or post-acne scars, would take at least three to six months, six weeks are good to begin with. Once you get into the routine, sow the seeds and reap the benefits, there will be no looking back.

How to Read This Book

Skin Rules presents a six-week plan to blemish-free, radiant skin. It does not cater to one symptom at a time. Right from identifying your skin type, skincare routine and skin treatments to changes in diet and lifestyle, the approach needs to be holistic. Let me unfold the plan for you week by week.

Week 1: This week is all about learning to know your skin. Often you are confused about your skin type. You don't know which products to use and what to include in your daily routine. Some people don't even have a daily ritual. They just use a random cold cream off the shelf. You need to prep your canvas if you want your creams to work their magic on your skin. Learn the correct art of cleansing and the right way to use moisturizers and sunscreens, which are armaments for your skin's defence.

Week 2: Imagine waking up to dull, lifeless skin every day. If you want a fresh start, do your skin a favour by removing all your make-up before hitting the bed the previous night. This week is about getting into the habit of removing your make-up every single day.

A lot of us are plagued with pimples, or at least whiteheads, at some point in our life. Many have flawless skin until the thirties and presto, enter the hormones to show how mighty they are and how they can inflict us with acne, open pores and cause blemishes at thirty. Discover ways to tackle pimples, sun spots, dark circles, dark lips, dark underarms—practically everything that leaves your skin dark.

One pimple or dark patch on your face and the world will be ready to give you advice. Some will be generous enough to tell you about a magic cream they used and how their dark spots vanished, not knowing that it was probably a harmful steroid. Others will give you remedies from the kitchen. And some will simply pour out their sympathies, pushing you further down the rabbit hole, as if this was the end of the world for you. Beware of all these benevolent advisers because there are too many fallacies and misconceptions floating around which could do you more harm than good. Sometimes things are accepted without raising eyebrows because they seem to make sense. For example, gulping down gallons of water and over-cleansing your gut will detox your skin . . . Now don't raise your eyebrows when I say both are not true. This week is also about avoiding common blunders and doing a reality check.

Week 3: This week is not about the CTM drill. It is about adding the icing to your cake of skincare. There is an influx of new skincare lines and anti-ageing lotions and potions. Amid this constant buzz, one may find it difficult to distinguish hype from reality. So get ready to feel confident when you walk down the beauty gallery and pick the most suitable serums and anti-ageing products for yourself.

Week 4: If you think rubbing a cream on your skin for six weeks is going to make you Prince Charming or Snow White, you are wrong. Your skin also needs nourishment from within. We are all aware that a healthy diet and exercise can help us beat diabetes, heart diseases, gut, kidney and liver issues. This week is to make you aware that food and exercise can also work wonders on your skin. We shall also discuss a few home remedies which have been passed down for generations and are good for your skin.

Week 5: This is probably the toughest week. It's about challenging your lifestyle. Your skin cells work overtime while you sleep, in order to overcome the agony they have undergone during the day. So when I say you need beauty sleep, it is not a fairy tale. Factors like pollution, stress, smoking, alcohol, sedentary hours in front of your computer are not only malignant for your internal organs, but also corrupt your skin. People feel meditation and yoga are only for spiritual seekers or the distraught. I say they are a way of life, a way of taking care of ourselves and respecting our body and our skin. So get ready for some serious mandates on skin and lifestyle. I'm sure you will thank me later.

Week 6: Do you wake up in the morning and look into the mirror to find some pits on your face, reminiscent of the acne you had when you were in high school? Do the red patches on your face or dryness on your body keep flaring up, ruffling your feathers way too often? Sometimes you cannot escape a dermatologist's appointment. This week is about seeking help from 'skin doctors'. It is also about understanding the pros and cons of various skin treatments rather than blindly following advertisements. New anti-ageing gizmos and skin-brightening gadgets are introduced every day.

The beauty and laser industries are growing bigger than one could have ever imagined. From gold-infused skincare to bee's venom, claims to make you younger or fairer are rising by the second. Indeed, there are age-defying innovations which help attain what was once considered impossible. But the credibility of these machines, lasers and treatments need to be researched before you sign up. This week, learn about what's latest in the field of cosmetic dermatology, what is really worth the buck and what is snake oil.

Now that the plan is made, it is time for execution. Mickey and I have pledged to work hard for the next six weeks. I invite you all to join us in our endeavour to achieve radiant skin. Follow your weekly skincare programme with passion, honesty, patience and enthusiasm.

WEEK 1

WEEK 1

1

Know Your Skin

'A journey of a thousand miles begins with a single step'

—Lao Tzu

Mickey had no clue about her skin type. She said her mother gave her good genes and so her skin did not need any extra care. 'Doc, why don't you tell me about all skin types if it is important. That way, I can help my family and friends buy the right products too. I want them all to glow on my big day.' Mickey was rather generous, I'd say. I sat with her for almost two hours, describing the various skin types.

When thirty-two-year-old Mrinal, an HR executive, went on the hunt for a night cream, she got thoroughly confused. There were a multitude of creams by innumerable brands. All of them looked tempting and promised miracles. But these creams were specially tailored for different skin types and would work best if we chose the right one. Mrinal's first hurdle was to identify her skin type. She sought help from the salesgirl at the desk. The salesgirl was sweet and helpful and Mrinal thought she had bought the best night cream for herself. However, within two days of applying the cream, she broke into a rash.

'I bought the cream the girl suggested!' she told me. What Mrinal didn't realize was that the salesgirl was neither a trained aesthetician nor a pharmacist. She was only selling her product. It is important to either consult a dermatologist or learn to identify your own skin type before buying a skincare product.

Like Mrinal, there are many people who do not know their skin type—and Mickey was no exception. There are many others who do not know what creams to buy for themselves. So let's start by learning to identify our skin type.

Know your skin

Skin is made up of the upper epidermis and lower dermis. The upper epidermis has many layers of cells. The topmost layers, composed of dead cells, lipids, keratin, urea, salts and 30 per cent water, together form the stratum corneum. They also make up the skin's natural moisturizing factors (NMF). The stratum corneum forms a barrier that protects the skin and prevents toxins from entering.

The epidermis consists of five layers. The lowermost layer of the epidermis, known as the stratum basale, is of significance to us. It comprises cells called keratinocytes and melanocytes. Keratinocytes form the factory that produces new cells. From this layer, old cells gradually travel upwards to reach the surface of the skin and are then shed in twenty-eight days. Melanocytes produce the pigment melanin that gives skin its colour.

The other layers

The lower part of skin is known as the dermis. The dermis contains an important molecule called hyaluronic acid—a polysaccharide glycosaminoglycan—that builds moisture in the skin. It has the unique capacity to bind and retain water molecules. It helps maintain the resilience and smooth texture of skin.

The dermis is also comprised of collagen fibres that give skin structural support and elastin fibres that give skin its suppleness and elasticity.

Sweat glands that secrete sweat, sebaceous glands (the oil glands of the skin) that secrete an oil called sebum, hair follicles (hair roots), blood vessels, lymphatics and nerves all lie in the dermis.

Below the dermis lies the subcutaneous or fat layer, followed by fascia, muscle and bone.

What does our skin do?

Apart from adorning us and making us look beautiful, our skin also forms the protective wall around our internal organs. It protects us against the scorching heat, the bitter cold, the swarm of microbes and the layers of pollution. It produces vitamin D. It acts like a warehouse which stores fat, water and metabolic products. It allows us to feel pain, touch, heat and cold. It also acts as a thermostat because it regulates temperature and protects us from too much cold or heat.

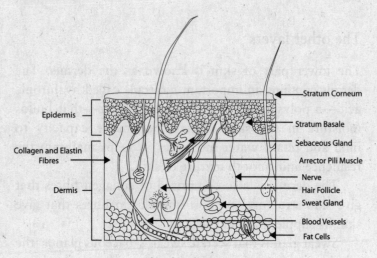

Epidermis

Collagen and Elastin Fibres

Dermis

Stratum Corneum

Stratum Basale

Sebaceous Gland

Arrector Pili Muscle

Nerve

Hair Follicle

Sweat Gland

Blood Vessels

Fat Cells

The skin diagram

Normal skin type

Normal oil and sweat production, a balanced moisture content of skin and a normal cell cycle with proper cell shedding together form normal skin.

You may not have flaky skin and your skin may not seem like an oil factory, but that does not mean you do not have to take care of it. You need as much skincare as a person with oily or dry skin.

How does one identify it?

- Normal skin is neither too dry nor too oily.
- The pores are barely visible.

- The skin is free of blemishes.
- The skin is smooth and radiant.
- There are hardly any imperfections.
- The skin does not react adversely to any product.

Causes

- Your genes!

How does one take care of it?

- Use a cleanser, moisturizer and sunscreen in the morning.
- Use a cleanser, an anti-ageing serum and a moisturizer at night.

Dry skin type

Skin that produces less sebum than normal skin is termed as dry skin. Normally, lipids, such as ceramides, cholesterol and fatty acids, present in the stratum corneum retain moisture and build a protective barrier against external agents. NMFs such as lactic acid, amino acid and urea help to bind in water. Dry skin lacks adequate lipids and NMFs, resulting in an impaired barrier function. This makes the skin more susceptible to allergies and dullness.

Skin loses water constantly, either by perspiration or through trans-epidermal water loss (TEWL). TEWL is the natural mechanism of passive water loss from the skin by diffusion from the deeper layers of the skin. Excessive perspiration or TEWL also increases dryness.

How does one identify it?

- The skin feels dry and rough to touch.
- There are no visible pores.
- The skin is less elastic.
- The skin appears lustreless and blotchy.
- The skin may be flaky and when you run your nails over it, it turns white.
- Fine lines may be visible.
- The skin may feel itchy.
- After washing your face, the skin feels stretched and tight.
- Extremely dry skin can result in calluses and cracks.

Causes

- Dry skin may be a result of your genetic composition. A result of which is that you have inherently less lipids in your skin and therefore your skin produces less oil.
- The oestrogen hormone can increase hyaluronic acid in the skin, to maintain fluid balance and structural integrity. During menopause, oestrogen is reduced, resulting in dryer skin.
- In people who suffer from hypothyroidism, the thyroid stimulating hormone (TSH) level is high. This can lead to dryness.
- Diabetes can also result in insulin alterations and dry skin.
- Just as the body goes through changes while ageing, so too does the skin. Chronological ageing occurs

as a natural process. The skin's ability to produce more collagen or hyaluronic acid or to retain lipids reduces due to cellular DNA damage. Hence, skin becomes drier and thinner. Extrinsic ageing is a result of external wear and tear and sun damage. Interestingly, this results in dry skin too. Water is lost from the keratinocytes in dry weather and during low temperatures, as in cold climates, leading to dry skin.

How does one take care of it?

Slather your skin with a rich moisturizer while it is slightly damp in order to trap the moisture. Look for ingredients such as shea butter, cocoa butter, vitamin E, squalene, coconut oil and geranium oil in your moisturizer. Use the moisturizer at least twice a day.

Most of the time, moisturizing adequately will solve the problem and reduce itchiness, flakiness, dull skin and fine lines.

Keep your baths short and do not bathe more than once a day. Being in the water for long hours causes the skin to dry as the skin cells are depleted of water in the bargain.

Bathe in cold or lukewarm water. Hot water evaporates easily from the skin and takes away the moisture, leading to dryness.

Use mild cleansing lotions or shower gels. Avoid soap bars. Soap alters the pH of the skin, changing it from acidic to alkaline. This, again, results in dryness.

Do not use scrubs and loofahs. Scrubbing can damage the lipid barrier layer of the skin and result in dryness.

Do not remain in an air-conditioned environment for long hours at a stretch. This dehydrates the skin. More so if you are sitting in front of the blower. Try to keep the temperature at 24–25° C if you are working in a centrally air-conditioned office. Take a ten-minute break and leave the air-conditioned room. Moisturize your skin at least thrice a day, once before leaving for work, once at bedtime and once during your lunch break at work.

Use a humidifier at home if you use room heaters in winter. Indoor heaters are as bad as air conditioners. They zap the moisture from the skin.

Wear gloves when working with detergents and solvents. Detergents and solvents damage the lipid layer of the skin.

Do not use alcohol-based toners and make-up removers. Alcohol strips moisture off the skin and increases dryness. Use oil-based make-up removers, balms, micellar water or rose water instead.

Do not use fruit or vegetable juices and packs on the skin. Remember, most fruit and vegetable juices are acidic. Acids can cause irritation and dryness of skin.

If you are undergoing treatments for acne or pigmentation, you may be given medicines and creams, both of which cause dryness. Isotretinoin, retinoic acid, glycolic acid, salicylic acid, adapalene and benzoyl peroxide will cause dryness. Chemical peels and some laser treatments may also do the same. Do not forget to balance the dryness with the help of moisturizers.

Anti-ageing creams with retinaldehyde or retinoic acid can also cause dryness. Use them thrice a week, alternating with a good hydrating cream containing hyaluronic acid. Make sure you use a sunscreen during the day.

Oily skin type

When sebaceous glands in our skin are hyperactive and produce excessive sebum, the skin is oily. The face and scalp are usually oilier than the rest of the body due to the concentration of sebaceous glands in these areas of the body.

Shoulders, chest and back can get oily too.

How does one identify it?

- The skin feels greasy all the time.
- There is oil on the face within an hour of washing. There are large pores on the surface of the skin.
- The skin is more prone to developing blackheads, whiteheads and large pimples.
- The skin looks shiny all the time.

Causes

- You may have inherited your parents' genes and so you have more oil glands in your skin, especially your face and scalp. So your skin produces more oil, typically on the face and scalp.
- Polycystic ovaries in females and increased dihydrotestosterone hormone in males can result in oily skin. Hormonal changes in the form of raised androgens during puberty will also result in oily skin.
- Stress can increase cortisol hormones leading to increased oil production in the skin.
- Certain medicines, such as steroids, can increase the oiliness of the skin.

How does one take care of it?

- Wash your face at least twice a day.
- Use a cleanser containing salicylic or glycolic acid at least once a day to unclog the pores and cleanse the skin.
- Use gel or matte sunscreens.
- Use water-based moisturizers.
- Do not use oil- or cream-based products on the skin. Look for products which say 'non-comedogenic'— this means they won't clog the pores.
- Avoid using milk, cream or high-fat yogurt on the skin.
- Strictly avoid popping your zits.
- Avoid scrubbing your face often. By doing so, you will strip the skin of its natural oils and damage the lipid layer protecting your skin. Also, the oil glands will produce more oil as a defence mechanism.
- Avoid massaging the skin. The oil glands will secret more oil when you do so.

Combination skin type

Combination skin comprises of an oily T-zone while the rest of the skin is either normal or dry. The oily T-zone is caused by an over-secretion of oil sebum. Lack of sebum or oil, and a corresponding lipid deficiency in the cheeks and chin cause dryness in the remaining parts. If the skin is normal in the cheeks and chin, it only means that there is adequate oil secretion in these areas.

How does one identify it?

- The skin feels normal or dry on the cheeks but is oily in the T-zone.
- Acne or blackheads occur on the forehead, nose and chin.
- Large pores are visible on the nose.
- T-zone is shiny.

Causes

- You have more oil glands in your T-zone. The rest of your face has an optimum number of oil glands.

'Bingo, that's my skin type, doc. I have blackheads on my nose all the time like black spots on my rather clear face,' said Mickey. So we crossed the first step. At least Mickey identified her skin type.

How does one take care of it?

- You will have to use a cleanser which is neither drying nor hydrating. A neutral soap-free cleanser works best. Avoid alcohol-based cleansers and toners.
- You could even use separate products for the oily and dry areas of the face.

Sensitive skin type

Sensitive skin is easily irritated by different factors, such as climate, skincare products and cosmetics, that are generally tolerated by normal skin.

The lipids in the upper stratum corneum of the skin are like the 'mortar' to the skin cells, which are the 'bricks'. Lipids provide permeability and stability and regulate fluids in the skin.

The effectiveness of skin lipids is dependent on enzyme activity, which is often weaker in sensitive skin. Thus, the protective function of the barrier is compromised in sensitive skin. This leads to excessive TEWL and allows irritants and toxins to penetrate the skin. The protection from chemicals, UV rays and pollutants is also compromised.

How does one identify it?

- The skin may turn red at the drop of a hat.
- There may be swelling, scaling, flaking, roughness or rashes.
- There may be itching, burning or a pricking sensation.
- One may develop a rash if there is a change in climate or environment.
- One may get eczemas too often.
- Most skincare products and cosmetics rarely suit people with sensitive skin.

Causes

- If one has genes where the lipids are deficient or defective from birth, one develops sensitive skin.
- In the case of females, hormone fluctuations due to the menstrual cycle, pregnancy and menopause can all affect the skin's resistance to irritants.

- Inadequate sleep and stress are both known triggers for sensitive skin.
- Low humidity, prevalent in centrally air-conditioned offices and in aeroplanes and central heating, dehydrates the skin and increases its sensitivity.
- Heat increases sweating and evaporation of moisture from skin. Cold climates dry the skin. Both can result in sensitive skin.
- UV radiation and environmental pollutants increase free radicals in the skin, weakening the natural defence mechanisms of the skin and making it sensitive.
- Creams, oils, lotions and cosmetics containing harsh chemicals, alcohol and preservatives can make the skin more sensitive by damaging the protective barrier layer of the skin.
- Fragrance is known to cause allergies in sensitive skin.
- Some surfactants that remove dirt can also remove skin lipids and harm the skin.
- Medicinal creams, especially steroids, damage the lipids, NMFs and keratin in skin and make it extremely sensitive.

How does one take care of it?

- Have a diet rich in antioxidants such as vitamins A, C and E and omega-3 fatty acids.
- Make sure to use sunscreen throughout the day.
- Avoid perfumes, deodorants and any other fragrance-based products.
- Do not forget to moisturize your skin at least twice a day.

- Avoid products with heavy synthetic dyes and harsh chemicals.
- Avoid products with alcohol and parabens.
- Stick to basic ingredients like aloe vera, coconut oil, glycerine, pantothenol, vitamin B5 and ceramides.
- Avoid wearing synthetic clothes.

'Just knowing your skin type is not enough,' I told Mickey. 'You also need to know about certain skin conditions and buy products accordingly. Let us run through them quickly.' From the corner of my eye, I could see her yawn but an incomplete tutorial was not an option for me.

The common skin conditions are:

Acne-prone skin

Gia tells me she has sensitive skin. I ask her what makes her say so. 'I get whiteheads with whatever cream or cosmetic I use,' she replies. My dear Gia, you do not have sensitive skin. You have acne-prone skin. Samir's doctor told him he had dry skin. But when he bought a moisturizer for dry skin, he developed whiteheads. So Samir should have ideally bought a product for dry, acne-prone skin.

Pigmented skin

Arin feels his skin is completely tanned. He has dark patches on his face and arms. The rest of his body is fair. This has been so for four to five years. Arin, a tan disappears within one and a half to three months. It does not remain for five years. You have developed pigmentation on the exposed parts of your body due to years of sun exposure.

Mature skin

Skin that is thin, dry, wrinkled, saggy and has a lot of blemishes and sun spots can be termed as mature or ageing skin. This is seen in people above the age of fifty-five.

My friend Marissa tells me her skin is weird. It gets oily sometimes and dry at other times. Well, Marissa, with age, your skin has been subjected to changes in climate, environment, medicines, creams, skin treatments and hormonal imbalances which can change the way it behaves.

Skin can also become dry as one ages. This is because the oil glands shrink in size with age and the lipid bilayer, which protects the skin, becomes thinner.

Skin also becomes thin due to the thinning of collagen and elastin fibres and damage of the lipid barrier layers of the skin.

'Hmm, so my mom and dad have mature skin now,' mumbled Mickey, beginning to understand the complexities of skin and its types.

Take a skin test

Step 1: Wash your face in the morning with a gentle cleanser.
Step 2: Pat it dry with a soft napkin and leave your skin bare.
Step 3: Do not apply anything on your skin for an hour.
Step 4: After an hour, take a tissue and spread it over your face evenly. Dab your skin.
Step 5: Look at the tissue and feel your skin as well.

If the tissue is clear, your skin is normal.

If the tissue has oil in the shape of a T, you have combination skin.

If the tissue is stained and oily, you have oily skin.

If the tissue has some fine flakes, you have dry skin.

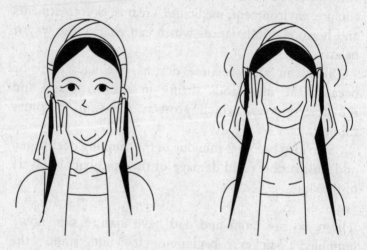

Tissue paper test

Identify your skin type

An hour after washing my face, my skin feels	An hour after washing my face, the tissue looks	My skin type is
Normal, not oily, not dry	Clear	Normal
Greasy and shiny	Blurred and smudged with oil	Oily
Tight and dry, sometimes flaky	Looks clear but sometimes tiny flakes are stuck to it	Dry
Feels greasy on the T-zone, the nose shines, the cheeks are normal or dry	An oily or smudgy area in the form of a T is seen	Combination

'Mickey, now keep in mind, you cannot use the same cream at all times. The cream you use will depend on your skin type, your skin condition and the climate you are in. Why don't you do a skin check for all your family members this week and identify their skin type? Trust me, you would be doing them a big favour.'

2

What Is Your Skin Telling You?

'Beauty is of the great facts in the world like sunlight, or springtime, or the reflection in dark water of that silver shell we call the moon'

—Oscar Wilde

'My skin is not too bad, doc, but my nails are chipping away to glory,' wailed Mickey.

'Mickey, nails can become weak due to frequent use of nail polish or nail polish remover containing acetone. Gel nails and artificial nails are indeed in vogue but too much exposure to UV rays can damage the nail. If you are in contact with chemicals constantly due to your profession and you often don't wear gloves, your nails can become brittle. If you have OCD and wash your hands with soap every other hour, your nails can become weak.'

'But, doc, I do none of that. No gel nails, no frequent washing, no chemicals. I fail to understand this. Help me, doc. I do want my natural nails to grow long so I can shape them well and apply a nail polish to match every outfit I wear for my various functions.'

'Mickey, do you know our skin often gives us signals about what is going on inside our body? We must learn to listen to our skin. And when I say skin, I mean nails and hair too because hair and nails are a part of skin. So, there is a hidden reason behind your brittle nails. Your nails are telling you that you are deficient in protein and biotin. Nails comprise of keratin, which is nothing but protein.'

Other deficiencies can also manifest as skin, hair or nail disorders. For example, if your knuckles are turning black, it's time to check if your vitamin B12 levels are low. If you develop dark circles despite sleeping well, your haemoglobin may be going down.

Skin is the largest organ of our body. We think of it simply as an outer covering of the body, like an orange peel, which we can abuse as we please. But it is a vital part of the body. It shields our internal organs, provides vitamin D, regulates body temperature and, most importantly, gives us signs of any internal problem.

We all look at ourselves in the mirror every day. Why not take a few moments to carefully examine our skin? To feel it and see if there is anything abnormal or different. Does it feel dry or oily? Does it look dull, oily or radiant?

If your skin feels dry, you have not moisturized it well. 'But I did apply a moisturizer before sleeping,' said a friend who works at a corporate office. You may have done so, but then you sat in your air-conditioned office for twelve hours. That is enough to dehydrate you. Your skin is asking for more. So please moisturize in the morning as well. My friend answered, 'I am in such a hurry in the morning. Where is the time to moisturize?'

Well, you could keep a bottle of moisturizer in your car and apply it on the way to work. If you travel by public transport, just keep one in your office drawer. You may be in the air-conditioning for long hours or in a place where the temperature is very low. This zaps the moisture from your skin and makes it dry. You need an extra amount of moisturizer. If you are using it only once a day, switch to twice a day now. And do not forget your arms, legs, hands, feet, neck and back.

If you suffer from frequent pimple outbreaks and are losing hair as well, it's time to find out if you have polycystic ovarian syndrome (PCOS) or raised androgens (male hormones which females also have in small quantities). This is an extremely common condition in girls who have attained menarche. Small cysts appear in the ovaries due to a hormonal imbalance in the body. This leads to a series of problems like acne, hair fall, hair growth on body parts like the face, weight gain and sometimes irregular periods. If you have any two of these symptoms, you should get an ultrasonography of your ovaries and do some blood tests during your menstrual cycle.

This will help you find out if you have PCOS or any other hormonal imbalance. If you happen to suffer from PCOS, make sure your weight is under control. And make sure you consult a gynaecologist. Sometimes all your efforts to treat acne will fail or you will end up doing twenty-odd sessions of laser hair removal and still suffer from disastrous pimples and hair growing on the body. But treat the PCOS—and lo and behold! Your acne will disappear, and so will your body hair suddenly respond to laser.

At a party one day, my friend said she was noticing some pigmentation on her back and arms. She was using double the amount of moisturizer and yet her skin felt dry. I asked her to get her blood tested for thyroid hormones. Sure enough, she had high levels of thyroid stimulating hormone (TSH). This signified that she was suffering from hypothyroidism. I asked her to consult an endocrinologist (a doctor who specializes in disorders of hormones). Hypothyroidism is an autoimmune disorder and it can cause dryness of skin and even pigmentation on the skin.

My father once developed pus-filled boils on his legs. I remember going to the local dispensary with him where Dr Singh told him that boils occur because of a bacterial infection called staphylococcus. 'You must be scratching your legs and your nails must be infected with bacteria,' he told my dad. I used to admire Singh Uncle. He was a doctor, after all. Something I would also be when I grew up.

'Oil your legs, they won't get dry and you won't keep scratching,' my granny would tell my dad. She was certainly not wrong. And she didn't have a post-graduate degree in skin to diagnose dry-skin woes. But that didn't work and Dad developed boils yet again. This time Singh Uncle asked dad to get his blood sugar tested. Dad was around thirty-five years old and he wouldn't believe that he could be suffering from diabetes at such a young age. But Singh Uncle was very strict. Dad couldn't possibly overrule his instructions. Besides, who would treat his wounds? So his blood tests were done. One blood sample was taken early in the morning after he fasted for twelve hours. Another blood sample was collected two hours after his lunch. Singh Uncle was in shock. Dad's reports showed that both his fasting and post-meal sugar levels were high. Singh Uncle must have cursed himself for not asking for these blood tests four months earlier, when Dad first got those boils. It happens with all doctors sometime or other. But all's well that ends well. At least the diagnosis was made. Dad was immediately put on anti-diabetic medicines and his wounds healed as if a genie had performed some miracle.

Diabetes can manifest in the form of bacterial infections like pus boils or itchy fungal rashes in the body folds. Sometimes wounds as simple as a scratch on the skin will either take ages to heal or be stubborn and just not heal. Sometimes there is excessive itching on the arms and legs without any visible skin rash. Another common condition seen both in diabetes and hypothyroidism is speckled pigmented patches over arms, legs and upper back. This condition, often mistaken as sun tan, is called cutaneous macular amyloidosis. It sometimes itches but most of the time it may be symptomless. 'Cutaneous' means skin, 'macular' means flat spots or patches, 'amyloidosis' means deposition of a protein-containing pigment called amyloid.

My friend Naina's nineteen-year-old son has a thick band of pigmentation on his neck. It looks like a layer of dirt. 'He doesn't bathe well, J, he is very unhygienic,' Naina said when she brought him to me one fine day after months of coaxing. The pigmentation didn't bother him as much as it bothered her. She had even scrubbed his neck a couple of times but the stubborn dirt did not budge. I told Naina that the stubborn dirt was not dirt at all. Darkening and thickening of skin, almost like thick rugosities on the neck, arms and armpits is known as acanthosis nigricans.

It is usually a sign of insulin resistance or diabetes. But it may also be seen in obese people.

One must get a blood test done to check both fasting and post-meal insulin levels as well as blood sugar levels to know if there is insulin resistance. Insulin resistance can eventually lead to diabetes. Insulin is a hormone produced by pancreas. It regulates the sugar level in the blood. Whatever sugar or carbohydrates we eat are utilized for energy with the aid of insulin. The excess sugar, however, is converted into fat. If you have insulin resistance, your cells do not respond to the insulin, and sugar gets accumulated in the blood, raising the blood sugar level. So it eventually leads to diabetes.

I get hives quite often. It is the body's way of fighting against something I am intolerant or allergic to. It could be allergy to food, pollen, fungi, dust, mites, etc. The condition is called urticaria. The only way to find out which one you are allergic to is by doing the skin allergy test or the prick test. However, if the allergy is acute and you have a lot of hives coming frequently, avoid doing the test. Your skin will be hyper-reactive in such a state and the test will show a lot of false results.

Finally, if you see a mole growing rapidly, you should get it tested. It could be heading towards skin cancer.

'Whoa, doc, the skin is indeed a mirror of what's going on inside our body,' said an amused Mickey.

'Yes, your skin is constantly trying to tell you something. Every mole, every dark or light spot, every growth tells you a story. It is like litmus paper telling you about a disease you may have. Do not ignore the messages your skin is relaying to you. Take your skin seriously.'

3

Your Skincare Ritual

'To accomplish great things, we must not only act,
but also dream; not only plan, but also believe'
—Anatole France

Mickey has no skincare routine. She uses any soap that
is lying on the shelf in her bathroom. On some days she
remembers to wash her face before going to sleep. On
other days, she grabs a bite and hits the sack as she is
too tired. She never uses moisturizers because she has
never felt the need. However, she makes sure she uses a
sunscreen on holidays. But she has a complaint. She still
comes back tanned. Does she reapply every two hours?
Most certainly not! And that's the catch, the reason behind
the sunscreen not working on most holidays. Having said
that, Mickey knew about the CTM (cleansing, toning,
moisturizing) routine.

'I am glad you are familiar with the CTM regime,
Mickey. But let me tell you, I like to do away with
toners. Toners are nothing but extended cleansers. They

are needed if you do not cleanse your skin well or do not manage to remove your make-up properly. You can completely do away with them unless you have extremely oily skin. If you have normal or dry skin, toners may actually increase dryness.'

I believe what our skin actually needs is the CHP (cleanse, hydrate, protect) ritual in the morning and the CCH (cleanse, correct, hydrate) ritual at bedtime. This means, in the morning, you clean with a cleanser, hydrate with a moisturizer and then protect with a sunscreen. You may apply make-up over your sunscreen.

At night, you must cleanse again. This means removing your make-up with a make-up remover, cleansing with a face wash and then, if your face still feels oily or clogged, using a toner or a scrub. Then you can apply a corrector. A corrector could be an anti-acne cream, a cream for pigmentation or an anti-ageing cream. Finish with a moisturizer for hydration.

Let us understand this regime in detail.

Cleansers

We don't realize the magnitude of particles that collect on our skin's surface at every moment. The stratum corneum of the skin sheds its cells daily. This is not visible to the naked eye. The skin produces sebum. This attracts dust which attaches to the skin's surface as dirt.

Cleansing

Cosmetics, creams, make-up, external pollutants, soot and grime can also settle on the skin and clog the pores.

There's so much for microorganisms to feast on, so don't you think cleaning all the muck is important? Cleansers remove all the dead cells, sweat, salts, grime, dirt, dust and make-up from the skin's surface, and help maintain skin hygiene.

Make sure to cleanse your face once in the morning and once at night. You must use the right kind of cleanser for your skin type.

When on the hunt for a cleanser, do not base your decision on the look of the cleanser, the fragrance or the packaging. Choose your cleanser based on your skin type and any existing skin condition such as acne. Also keep in mind the climate.

Normal skin

A cleanser that leaves your skin feeling fresh and clean is all you need. You can choose any cleanser for normal skin, from Himalaya to LaMer. You can even use syndet bars. Syndet bars are synthetic detergent-based cleansers that contain less than 10 per cent of soap and typically have a more neutral/acidic pH (5.5–7), similar to the pH of normal skin.

Some examples of face washes for normal skin:

- Crème Lavante face wash
- Saslic foaming face wash
- Sebamed liquid face and body wash
- Episoft cleansing lotion

Dry skin

If your skin feels dry all the time, you should use a gentle cleanser. It should have added moisturizers and super fatty acids such as petrolatum, lanolin, mineral oil, cocoa butter, glycerine, shea butter and ceramides. Natural ingredients like jojoba oil, aloe vera, coconut oil, soybean oil and olive oil are also found in cleansers for dry skin. These cleansers clean the skin and leave a thin film of moisture on the surface, giving it a supple feel. If you have dry skin, you should avoid antibacterial soaps. They will indeed keep your skin germ-free but will also make it dry. Avoid cleansers with exfoliants such as salicylic or glycolic acid. Also avoid using basic soaps on facial skin. Basic soaps have a high pH and are irritating to the skin as a result of their damaging effects on the skin barrier.

Some examples of face washes for dry skin:

- A-Derma soothing foaming gel
- Cetaphil gentle skin cleanser
- D-wash face wash
- Sebamed olive face and body wash

Oily skin

An oily face can be very annoying, especially when you have meetings, presentations or outdoor work. 'I can fry an egg on my face, do something, doc,' is a common phrase most people use when they come to me with oily skin. Oily skin is prone to acne, both blackheads and whiteheads. This is a result of androgen hormones which signal the oil glands to produce oil (sebum) in excess. There is no need to get frustrated. Let us first pick the perfect cleanser for you. Choose a cleanser or face wash that foams gently. Too much foam can be harsh on the skin while a little foam will remove the oil and leave the skin free from any greasy residue. You can use a cleanser with salicylic acid in it to help unclog the pores. Botanicals such as aloe vera or tea tree oil balance oil production and support clarity. Alpha hydroxyl acid, such as glycolic acid or lactic acid, present in cleansers will help to gently exfoliate skin and can be used too.

However, your cleanser should not leave your skin feeling dry and tight. So make sure your cleanser does not have alcohol in it.

Some examples of face washes for oily skin:

- Sebamed clear face foam face wash
- Sebium gel moussant
- Ahaglow advanced face wash
- Saslic face wash

Combination skin

A cleanser for combination skin must be neither extremely moisturizing nor too drying. Alternatively, one can use a face wash for oily skin on the T-zone and a face wash for dry skin on the rest of the face.

Some examples of face washes for combination skin:

- Hyséac cleansing gel
- Cetaphil oily skin cleanser
- Episoft OC cleansing gel
- Ethiglo face wash

Acne-prone skin

Mallika says she cannot use any face wash or cream. Whenever she does, she breaks out. She has acne-prone skin. Those with acne-prone skin should use antibacterial cleansers. They help decrease the load of Propionibacterium acne, a particular microbe which causes acne or pimples. Salicylic acid-based cleansers unclog pores and reduce oiliness. They are a very good option for those who tend to break out easily.

If you are on any oral medication or topical creams for acne, such as isotretinoin, tretinoin, retinol, adapalene, benzoyl peroxide or even chemical peels, antibacterial or salicylic cleansers should be avoided. They can irritate and dry up the skin. So gentle cleansing with a non-soap cleanser (names mentioned in face washes for sensitive skin) is important for this group of patients.

Some examples of face washes for acne-prone skin:

- FCL Alpha Beta acne cleanser
- Acmed face wash
- D'acne face wash
- Avene cleanance gel

Sensitive skin

Do you develop a rash with any face wash you pick off the shelf? You need a cleanser for sensitive skin. I would advise you to stick to medicated ones. Stay away from the fancy, fragranced face washes, however chic they may seem. You should look for a cleanser with zero fragrance and alcohol. It should be neutral to acidic pH and have emollient properties, to keep the stratum corneum hydrated. Micellar water is best for sensitive skin. Micellar water is a mixture of thermal waters which are rich in minerals and have skin-healing properties, non-ionic surfactants, which are not harsh on the skin unlike soaps, and some form of glycerine to keep the skin soft. Micellar water absorbs all dirt and impurities and cleanses the skin thoroughly. It does not lather or change the skin pH. Hence, people with sensitive skin now have a cleanser to look forward to without having to worry about the perils of a face wash or a cleanser.

Some examples of face washes for sensitive skin:

- Sebamed olive face and body wash
- Bioderma Sensibio H_2O micelle solution
- Uriage Thermal Micellar Water
- Aquaderm face and body wash

Now let us look at the other forms of cleansers available in the market.

Scrubs

Scrubs help remove lodged dirt through abrasive physical action imparted by natural or synthetic particulate ingredients. Natural particles include fruit seeds (e.g. peach, apricot or apple), nut shells (e.g. walnut or almond), grains (oats, wheat), sandalwood and sugar. Synthetic particles include polyethylene or polypropylene beads and aluminium oxide or sodium tetraborate decahydrate granules. They help in mechanical skin exfoliation and remove dead skin cells. Of these, aluminium oxide and fruit pits are the most abrasive. Their sharp edges may lead to irritation for those with dry or sensitive skin.

Those with normal skin and oily skin can use scrubs once a week to exfoliate and unclog pores.

Cleansing creams

As the name suggests, they cleanse and moisturize. Therefore, they are better suited for dry skin. They can contain wax, mineral oil, petrolatum or detergents such as borax. Long lasting oil-based make-up can be effectively removed with these cleansers.

Cleansing milk and lotions

They are the water-based counterparts to cleansing creams. They can be used to remove water-based make-up with a cotton ball or a wipe. They can also be rinsed off with water.

Toners

They are best suited for oily, acne-prone skin and areas like the T-zone that produce excess sebum. They are also used to remove make-up. They can be applied directly to target areas with a cotton ball or a tissue. It is better to avoid alcohol-based toners. Rosewater or any micellar water is a better option than a harsh menthol– or camphor-based toner. Those with dry or sensitive skin need not use toners at all.

Motorized brushes

Motorized brushes, such as clarisonic brushes, have become popular as home skincare tools. They are battery-operated brushes with bristles that move back and forth in a circular motion. The bristles help remove make-up and dirt from the skin's surface. They are a good option for those who work outdoors, sweat a lot or use a lot of make-up. People with normal, oily or combination skin can use them. Those with dry or sensitive skin should avoid using them.

Face packs

Packs made of fuller's earth, fruit extracts and green clay are known to reduce oil from the skin's surface. Fuller's earth, or *multani mitti*, can be mixed with rosewater and applied on the face. It should be left on for about ten minutes and then rinsed off. It can be used once a week. Those with dry or sensitive skin should not use this. Some face packs contain sea mud and algae, and are said to have anti-ageing benefits. They are better suited for mature skin, to prevent fine lines and reduce pores. They can be mixed with water or honey and then applied on the skin. Those with sensitive skin should not use any packs.

Masks

I am amazed at the number of pictures of charcoal masks that flood my Instagram. Charcoal masks are said to kill germs, remove oil from the skin and clean the skin thoroughly. The mask contains charcoal and a kind of glue. It is applied to the entire face and neck and allowed to dry for fifteen to twenty minutes. The mask is then pulled off. The pulling action removes fine hairs too, leaving the skin smooth and radiant. However, if used too often, the skin's natural lipids may get damaged and result in rashes or itchy skin. Do not use these masks if you have dry or sensitive skin.

The other masks that are quite popular are the skin-brightening masks, which contain ingredients such as arbutin, bearberry, niacinamide, liquorice and other botanical extracts known to lighten the skin. They brighten up the skin temporarily and are great to be used before a party. They are usually safe for all skin types. However, those with sensitive skin must always use masks with caution.

Yet another mask that floods the current market is the gel sheet mask made popular by the Koreans. These are left on the skin for twenty to thirty minutes, during which the solution in the mask gets soaked into the skin and brightens it. There is no added benefit. Honestly, it is just another before-party mask.

Have you heard of sleepover masks? You actually apply them on the skin and leave them overnight, allowing the active ingredients to gradually get absorbed into the deeper skin layers, working their way towards cleansing and brightening the skin.

Ingredients you could look out for if you have oily skin are charcoal and clay. If you have dry skin, look for glycerine, hyaluronic acid and aloe vera in your mask.

If you have sensitive skin, I'd say it is best to avoid using any masks available in the shops. Instead make your own mask without using lemon or tomato or any fruit containing citric acid, which can irritate the skin further. Look up chapter 14 for some safe DIY masks.

Moisturizers

Why do we need to moisturize at all? Let us understand the skin better to be able to answer this.

The stratum corneum has cells which overlap to form a protective barrier. There is also a lipid bilayer which comprises free fatty acids, cholesterol and ceramides.

In addition, the cells have NMFs which are made up of amino acids, urocanic acid and minerals. All these together have the ability to retain water in the epidermis and limit the loss of NMFs, as well as loss of water from the skin, through TEWL. Cold weather, low temperatures, air conditioners, room heaters, lack of humidity, steam, sauna, bubble baths, hot-water showers, bar soaps, foaming washes and scrubs all strip the lipids from the skin, disrupting the skin barrier.

In order to replenish the lost water and prevent the skin from becoming dry and flaky, we need to moisturize.

Always apply a moisturizer on slightly damp skin, ideally within three to five minutes of your bath or washing your face. This locks the moisture within the skin and keeps it hydrated.

How do you know which moisturizer is good for your skin type? Well, this might help.

Normal skin

You can use a moisturizing cream for your face and a lotion for your body. Moisturize at least once a day.

Oily skin

Opt for lotions or water-based moisturizers. Look for lactic acid as an ingredient. It has both exfoliating and hydrating properties. Dimethicone and hyaluronic acid are great ingredients too. My patient Chris has very oily skin and hates using creams, especially when it is hot. I gave her the option of using sunscreen in the day and skipping the moisturizer. I also gave her a lightweight hyaluronic acid–based lotion for the night. What she really loved was the micellar water that I had asked her to use during the day when she was sweaty. She felt refreshed each time she sprayed the water on her face, her make-up stayed put and her skin felt hydrated.

Dry skin

You should choose a cream as it has more oil and will hydrate better. Use a thicker cream at night. Remember, the greater the oil content, the better the absorption through the barrier layer of the skin and the moisturization. Look for ingredients like dimethicone, hyaluronic acid, glycerine, vitamin E, shea butter, cocoa butter and squalene. If your skin is extremely dry and flaky, you should use an ointment base at bedtime. While a moisturizer gets absorbed, an ointment leaves a much-needed oily film on the skin surface. You must moisturize at least twice a day in summer and thrice a day in winter.

Combination skin

Use a light moisturizing cream or lotion. Moisturize at least once a day. 'This is for you, Mickey,' I emphasized.

Sensitive skin

Avoid using essential, aromatic oils. Stick to fragrance-free creams or natural oils like coconut, safflower or almond. Oil your skin at least twice a day.

Mature skin

Now this is not really a skin type but I'd like to mention it because people above the age of fifty usually develop dryness. The skin becomes thinner and wrinkled. So you need heavy moisturizers. If your moisturizer has hyaluronic acid or olive oil or coconut oil in it, it's the right one for you.

Common concerns about moisturizers

'I have oily skin but it becomes dry every time I go to Germany on my business trips,' says Mihir. Like Mihir, a lot of you must be getting confused trying to figure out your skin type. You must remember that the temperature of your surrounding impacts your skin. So if you go to places which have cold, dry climate, you will need a thicker moisturizer than what you normally use on a day-to-day basis. If it is hot and humid, you should either use a lightweight moisturizer or a gel formulation.

Forty-nine-year-old Kashmira had never used a moisturizer as she felt her skin was always oily. But her skin was now becoming dry and she didn't know what to use. Like Kashmira, each and every one of us will face this issue as we age. Don't forget: as we age, our skin ages too. The skin becomes dry as the epidermis becomes thinner, the lipids are lost and the sebaceous glands secret less oil. Hormones also change. Lack of oestrogen makes the skin dry and dull. So we will need to moisturize more often, use thicker creams and avoid hot-water showers and soaps which can dehydrate the skin.

Trisha said her face was oily but the skin on the rest of her body was very dry. This is quite possible. A moisturizer that is suitable for one's face need not suit their body. In such cases, you will need to use different moisturizers for the face and body. When you go to buy a moisturizer, you must know a little bit about the ingredients in order to choose the right one.

The three types of moisturizers are emollients, humectants and occlusives.

An emollient increases the water content of the stratum corneum and makes it supple and soft. The effect of an emollient lasts for four to five hours. Emollients have an anti-inflammatory effect, so they repair the skin. They also reduce itching and have a soothing effect on inflamed or damaged skin. Dimethicone, cyclomethicone, castor oil, jojoba oil, propylene glycol, octyl stearate, isopropyl palmitate and isostearyl alcohol are some examples of emollients.

Humectants such as glycerine, hyaluronic acid, sodium hyaluronate, sodium PCA, propylene glycol and heparan sulphate attract water and add moisture to the skin. Glycerine also modulates aquaporins, which are the water channels in the skin. It is a good ingredient to look for in a moisturizer. Hyaluronic acid is another great ingredient as it has the ability to attract and retain more than 1000 times its weight in water. It plumps up the skin and helps in new collagen formation. It also gives the temporary appearance of smoother skin with fewer wrinkles.

A word of caution regarding humectants: In dry weather they can suck the moisture from within the skin. So always pick moisturizers which contain both occlusives and humectants.

Occlusives are oily substances that coat the skin and prevent water from evaporating from the surface. They function like a plastic wrap that protects food and form a shield only as long they are there. When the occlusive is washed off, its effect is gone. The skin will lose its moisture due to evaporation and become dehydrated. Oils, lanolin, stearyl alcohol, cetyl alcohol, lecithin, squalene, mineral oil, petrolatum and silicones are occlusives. Mineral oils have been used for many years. However, industrial mineral oil was found to be carcinogenic. And petroleum jelly, when tested, had some amount of petroleum distillates. Hence, a lot of manufacturers do not use mineral oil and petrolatum any more and instead opt for natural ingredients such as shea butter, cocoa butter, sesame seed oil, etc.

There are various fatty acids that repair the skin barrier. I love palmitic acid, found in palm oil, and stearic acid, found in shea butter. These oils help to repair the skin barrier and keep the skin hydrated. Your skin barrier can also be repaired by taking omega-3 fatty acid supplements, evening primrose oil, fish oil, borage seeds, flax seeds and salmon.

Mustard oil can irritate the skin. Those of you who are fond of oils need to pick the correct ones for yourself. Borage seed oil, safflower seed oil and jojoba oils aid in skin barrier repair as they have anti-inflammatory properties. Apricot kernel seed oil and cranberry seed oil are doing the rounds now as they are rich sources of essential fatty acids. They can be taken orally and applied on the skin as well.

Frieda wanted to know if she and her husband could use the same moisturizer. Honestly, men do not need heavy moisturizers. Men's sebaceous glands secrete more oil. And men do not use numerous cosmetics on their skin or indulge in many facial treatments. Hence there is minimal trans-epidermal water loss. What men need is an emollient which makes the skin soft and smooth. Dimethicone is the most preferred ingredient. It is found in creams and after-shave lotions. However, men with dry skin eczemas or atopic dermatitis need thicker moisturizers. Females need a combination of occlusives, emollients and humectants. Not just to moisturize and protect their skin, but also to prevent fine lines and wrinkles which appear due to dryness.

Some medicated moisturizers contain lactic acid or urea. Lactic acid and urea increase the water-holding capacity of the skin and also act as mild exfoliants. Look for these ingredients when you have calluses, thick dead flaky skin or cracks on the soles of your feet.

	Normal skin	Dry skin	Oily skin	Sensitive skin	Mature skin
Type of moisturizer	Water-based, non-greasy, silicone-based	Heavier oil–based	Water-based, non-comedogenic	With soothing ingredients, i.e. aloe, chamomile	Petroleum-based with antioxidants or alpha hydroxy acids
Number of applications	Once or twice a day	Three to four times a day	At least once a day	Twice a day	At least twice a day
Examples	Cetaphil moisturising cream, Ictyane HD cream, Elovera cream	Venusia moisturising cream, Cetaphil DAM cream, Hydromax moisturizing cream	Emolene cream, Rheacalm light cream, Sebamed clear care gel	Epitheliale AH cream, Sebamed moisturizing cream, Hyalugel plus cream	Maxrich intensive moisturizing cream. Ureadin fusion melting cream, Venusia max cream

Restoring your pH balance

Normal skin has an acidic pH of around 5 to 5.5. This pH is maintained by the acid mantle of the skin. It forms a protective barrier, blocking harmful bacteria, micro-organisms and toxins and restoring moisture to the skin. Dry skin has an alkaline pH, i.e. pH above 7. Hence it is more sensitive and prone to allergies and eczemas. pH-balanced products help restore the acid mantle and the protective lipid layer of the skin. They are available in the form of moisturizers and aid in repairing dry, flaky skin, and even skin wounds. Soaps and detergents make the skin more alkaline and increase dryness.

Sunscreens

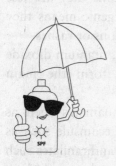

Sun protection

Sunscreens are products which prevent ultraviolet rays from being absorbed by the skin. They are available in the form of creams, gels, lotions, sprays and now even capsules.

Let us first understand these rays. Solar radiation comprises UV rays, visible light and infrared rays.

UV rays that reach the earth's surface comprise UVA (320–400nm) and UVB (290–320 nm) rays. Visible rays are at about 400–800 nm and infrared rays are anything above 800 nm.

Wavelengths less than 320 nm are absorbed by the upper layers of the skin, namely the stratum corneum and the epidermis. Wavelengths greater than 320 nm enter the deeper part of the skin, the dermis. All rays cause the breakdown of cell membrane, lipids, structural proteins and DNA of the skin.

Exposure to UVA rays can cause suntan, wrinkles, pigmentation, sun spots and even skin cancer.

UVB rays are responsible for sunburns and skin cancer. Visible rays and infrared rays are said to increase pigmentation (any dark patches on the skin). To protect the skin from all these rays, we need to use a sunscreen every single day.

Always look for sunscreens which say 'broad spectrum, non-comedogenic, hypoallergenic'. Broad spectrum means they offer protection from both UVA and UVB rays. Non-comedogenic means they are less likely to cause whiteheads. Hypoallergenic means they are less likely to produce allergic reactions or rashes.

Physical ingredients are zinc oxide, titanium dioxide and iron oxide. These ingredients form the main constituents of mineral sunscreens.

Safe chemical ingredients are cinnamates such as octinoxate, octyl methoxy cinnamate; ecamsule such as mexoryl, benzophenones, avobenzone; anthranilates such as methyl anthranilate; and salicylates such as octisalate, homosalate.

For best results, opt for a sunscreen which has both physical and chemical sunscreen ingredients. Some of the newer ones even protect from infrared rays. So if you are cooking most of the time or exposed to harsh indoor lights, use these sunscreens which protect from visible light and infrared rays as well as from UVA and UVB rays.

Now it's time to understand the SPF game.

SPF or sun protecting factor is a measure of protection from UVB rays. A higher SPF is recommended for Caucasian skin as it is more prone to skin cancer.

Table 1

SPF	Proportion of UVB blocked (per cent)
15	93
20	95
30	96.7
40	97.5
50	98.3

For Indian skin types, it is essential to look at the PA value which indicates protection from UVA rays.

Table 2

PA	Protection from UVA rays
+	Fair
++	Moderate
+++	Good
++++	Excellent

For regular use, one should opt for a sunscreen with SPF 30 and PA +++

If you have dry skin, use a cream-based sunscreen. And if you have oily skin, use a gel-based or matte sunscreen. For larger surface areas, use a lotion or a spray.

Having said that, the effect of even the best sunscreen will last for only two hours if outdoors. Ideally, therefore, it should be reapplied every two hours. And more frequently during outdoor activities when you sweat.

How much sunscreen should one apply?

The current US Food and Drug Administration (FDA) standard recommends 2 mg/cm^2 of skin surface. Remember to apply it on the back of your neck, ears and hairline.

Table 3

Face and neck	½ teaspoon (3 ml) of sunscreen
Each arm	½ teaspoon (3 ml) of sunscreen
Each leg	1 teaspoon (6 ml) of sunscreen
Feet	1 teaspoon on both feet
Chest	1 teaspoon
Back	2 teaspoons to full back

The most common questions asked about sunscreens:

1. *'My grandma never used sunscreen, yet her skin is flawless,' said Kriti when I asked her to apply sunscreen every day.*

Kriti, our grandparents were living in a better environment. The air was less polluted and the ozone layer wasn't as depleted as it is now.

2. *Sunscreens are so sticky, I cannot use them.*

Not any more. The market is flooded with new easy-to-use sunscreens that are not greasy. Ask your dermatologist or refer to the table at the end of this chapter.

3. *Sunscreens make my face look white.*

The older sunscreens made the skin look chalky and white. Zinc oxide and titanium dioxide, essential physical ingredients in a sunscreen, were responsible for this. Haven't you seen cricketers paint their faces white? This is zinc oxide, the best barrier from sun rays. However, one can't wear a white mask and go out on a regular basis. But now, zinc oxide and titanium dioxide are broken into micronized nanoparticles and incorporated into sunscreens. So you get the benefits without the white look.

4. *I break out when I use sunscreen.*

You are not using the appropriate sunscreen. Choose a gel-based sunscreen or a matte one with ecamsule. Oil or cream-based sunscreens can clog your pores, causing blackheads and whiteheads. Look for sunscreens which say 'non-comedogenic', 'gel', 'oil-free', 'dry touch', 'for acne-prone skin' or 'matte finish'.

Matte finish sunscreens contain silicones that ensure the pores are not clogged. They also reduce oil secretion and stickiness. They are best suited for people with oily skin.

Water-resistant sunscreens are occlusive and may clog pores. Avoid using them. Do not wear sunscreen for long hours if you tend to break out. If you work indoors and have no exposure to rays, you may wash your face an hour after reaching your office.

5. *My skin turns dark when I use sunscreen.*

All you have to do is change your sunscreen. Avoid ingredients such as avobenzone and titanium dioxide in your sunscreen. Sometimes you may be allergic to these ingredients. Using these could result in darker skin.

6. *I don't step out into the sun; I just sit in my car and reach office. Why should I use a sunscreen?*

UVA rays penetrate the glass in automobiles. Laminated glass used on windows offers some UV protection. However, rear side windows are made of non-laminated glass and transmit a significant amount of UVA rays. For adequate UV protection, all your car windows should have dark, protective UV shields which are available as laminated or tinted glass or film. However, as per traffic regulations, these tinted glasses are no longer allowed unless you have special permission. So the bottom line is that even if you travel by car, your skin still needs sunscreen.

Similarly, if you are working in chic glass buildings which do not have curtains, you are being exposed to UVA rays.

My friend Karishma loves to sit by her French windows on Sunday mornings and sip her coffee. She is indoors, yet she gets exposed to UV rays. So she does need a sunscreen, even at home. My aunt thinks she has zero sun exposure as she is a homemaker and does not step out of the house during the day. So she doesn't use a sunscreen. What she doesn't realize is that she is exposed to sun rays while making her trip to the balcony to water her plants, to the terrace to dry wet clothes and to the bus stop to wait for her kid's school bus. The short walk from our car to the office door or a walk to the café next door during a break is enough to do the damage.

7. *Aditi is an actor and feels that her make-up has enough SPF.*

Foundation make-up provides SPF 3 to 4, because of its pigment content, for up to four hours after application. BB creams offer up to 40 per cent of the sun protection claimed by them. It is always better to wear a sunscreen first and then layer on make-up that has SPF. There are tinted sunscreens and sunscreens with primers available. These allow the make-up to blend well without making the skin appear patchy.

8. *Ashfaq says he doesn't like to use a sunscreen because his face becomes sweaty on applying a sunscreen.*

Sunscreens which have more chemical ingredients change UV rays into heat. This causes sweat. To avoid this problem, opt for sunscreens with more physical ingredients like titanium dioxide and zinc oxide.

9. *Marissa recently had a fabulous holiday in the Alps where it was snowing heavily. Yet, she came back tanned.*

Snow reflects 80 per cent of the sun's rays; sand reflects 25 per cent and 80 per cent of the UVA rays that pass through clouds. So you must apply a sunscreen even on a cloudy day or when it is snowing. Remember to apply your sunscreen on all the exposed parts of your body.

Physical protection helps a lot when outdoors. Full-length trousers, long skirts, full-sleeved shirts and kurtis provide protection from UV rays. If you tend to tan or pigment easily, it is advised that you wear such clothes. Clothes made from tightly woven fabric offer better protection than loose ones. Also, darker-coloured clothes offer better sun protection than lighter ones. Wide-brimmed hats, umbrellas and scarves can also be used when outdoors.

10. *Rishabh says he leaves for work before 10 a.m. when the sun is not very bright. So he doesn't apply a sunscreen.*

Well, Rishabh, you are only partly correct. UVB rays are most intense between 10 a.m. and 4 p.m. However, as long as you see daylight, UVA rays are present with a fairly constant intensity. So there is no such 'safe time' unless it is before sunrise or after sunset.

11. *How will I get my vitamin D if I don't step out in the sun?*

This is a common question. Most people get more than enough vitamin D through regular, incidental sun exposure. And even if you always wear sunscreen, some UVB rays will still penetrate your skin, stimulating vitamin D production. Furthermore, after a limited amount of sun exposure, vitamin D production reaches its maximum and stops. UV exposure beyond this actually breaks down vitamin D.

The US FDA recommends a balanced diet and a daily 600 IU vitamin D3 supplement, along with 1 g calcium to obtain adequate vitamin D. A diet rich in vitamin D includes fortified milk, cereals, mushrooms, eggs, liver, cod liver oil and fish such as salmon, tuna and mackerel.

12. *Rimi's seven-year-old plays soccer and she feels he has turned two shades darker.*

This is the effect of UV rays. Sunscreen can be applied on children above the age of six months. It is advisable to plan indoor activities between 11 a.m. to 3 p.m. Avoid sun exposure during these hours because rays are the harshest at this time. It also helps to be fully clothed. Caps and hats should be worn. Preferably, use a physical sunscreen with SPF 15. Make sure to use a sunscreen before and after a swim or an outdoor sport.

Oral sunscreens: Supplements containing polypodium leucotomos, β-carotene, lycopene, vitamin C (ascorbate), vitamin E (tocopherol), nicotinamide, afamelanotide, grape seed extract and ubiquinone are known to protect the skin from visible light and infrared rays. Visible light is known to increase facial pigmentation, such as melisma, and sun-induced pigmentation. Infrared rays cause the skin to age by reducing skin elasticity and firmness and facilitating wrinkle formation.

Further photo protection can be achieved by applying a facial foundation. Facial foundation contains iron oxide, zinc oxide and kaolin, all of which block UV rays. Many of them now contain organic sunscreens as well, using octyl methoxycinnamate and oxybenzone, to provide an SPF rating.

Facial powders, applied on top of the facial foundation, provide even more sun protection. They allow the facial foundation to remain in place, while coating the skin with an additional layer of kaolin, talc and iron oxide. Powders are also excellent at absorbing sweat and sebum that can destroy the facial foundation film and literally float the photo protection right off your face. The face powder can be dusted with a loose brush over the facial foundation that has been applied over the sunscreen-containing moisturizer. Never forget to wear a hat, scarf, umbrella and big sunglasses, in addition to cosmetics, to protect yourself from the sun.

Skin type	Examples of sunscreen
Normal	Avene VHP SPF50 Sunscreen, UV Smart Daily Sunscreen, Sebamed Multi Protect Sun Cream
Oily	La Shield lite, Isdin Fotoprotector Gel, Suncros Matte Finish Soft Gel
Dry	Sebamed Sunscreen Lotion, Shadowz SPF 50, Rivela Sunscreen Lotion
Combination	Avene Dry Touch, Photostable sunscreen, Suncros Tint
Sensitive	Isdin Fusion water, Coola Mineral sunscreen, Z Block Sunscreen
For swimming	Suncros Aquagel, Neutrogena Beach Defense, Isdin Fotoultra Unify Lotion

Now Mickey has clearly understood what her skincare ritual should be. I hope you all have too.

4

Acquainting Yourself with Labels

'Genes and family may determine the foundation of
the house, but time and place determine its form'
—Jerome Kagan

Every time Mickey's sister is at an international airport,
she cannot resist the temptation to buy a range of
skincare products. However, the products only adorn
her dressing table because she doesn't know how to use
them or finds the labels difficult to understand. Mickey
thinks it's a complete waste of money and I agree with
her. Once you know what the labels on these products
mean, you will be able to buy your basic skincare
products easily and not end up wasting money on those
that don't suit you.

I shall help you get familiar with some common terms
and labels.

1. Normal skin, oily skin, dry skin, combination skin,
   sensitive skin: This has been described already and

it only means the product is apt for the skin type mentioned on the label.

2. Hypoallergenic: This means the manufacturer claims that there are less chances of an allergy with this product. However, this does not mean that the product is sure not to cause any rashes or allergies.

3. Non-comedogenic: A comedone is a whitehead or a blackhead in medical jargon. Non-comedogenic indicates that the product does not cause comedones. People with oily or acne-prone skin could use this product. However, it does not completely stop acne from occurring. US FDA does not define any ingredient as non-comedogenic or hypoallergenic. And there aren't any standardized tests to determine whether a product is really hypoallergenic or non-comedogenic. But referring to these labels will at least give you some direction.

4. Date of manufacturing and date of expiry: This doesn't need explanation but please do not be stingy and use products way past their expiry date just because you spent a bomb on them. Check the date of manufacturing and the date of expiry. If the date of expiry is close and you think you won't be able to finish using the cream, do not buy it. Once a product crosses the date of expiry, its quality begins to deteriorate.

5. PAO: This stands for 'period after opening'. Some skincare products and cosmetics carry a PAO symbol (a number followed by an M and an open jar icon). The PAO tells you when the product needs to be thrown away once opened. For example, a '6M' would mean you should discard the product six months after you

have opened it. Again, this is not 100 per cent reliable but it is better to follow it.

6. Fragrance-free: Manufacturers are allowed to call their products fragrance-free if the ingredients are not included only for the sake of emitting an aroma. However, some fragrant ingredients are used as preservatives or just to give a cosmetic effect to the product and the product can still be called fragrance-free.

7. Preservative-free: Do not go by this term. A preservative is used to protect just about any product from mould and bacteria. Any product with water in it has to have a preservative as well, otherwise it is sure to decay. Do not be afraid of preservatives. There are many natural preservatives such as vitamins, turmeric, rosemary, thyme, oregano, salts, silver citrate, potassium sorbate and essential oils that can be used safely in products. Products with natural preservatives can last for up to a year. Synthetic preservatives such as isothiazolones, urea derivatives, halogen-organic actives and EDTA are safer than parabens.

8. Paraben-free: Parabens have been the most common preservatives in any product since the 1950s due to their excellent antibacterial and antifungal properties. However, it was found that parabens mimic the hormone oestrogen by binding to oestrogen receptors. It was thus hypothesized that the use of paraben-based products could cause early puberty, breast cancer and low fertility in males. It has since been proven that for parabens to have effects similar to oestrogen, the dose of the preservative has to be 25000 times more than what is currently used in a preservative. And the link

between parabens and breast cancer has also been discredited due to insufficient scientific evidence. Nonetheless, the concentration of propylparaben and butylparaben is limited to 0.4–0.14 per cent in products manufactured in Europe. It has also been banned in diaper products. US FDA has claimed that the current low amounts used as preservatives are safe. There is no cumulative effect of parabens used over a period of time. The percentage used is so small that it gets washed away with cleansing. However, some people are allergic to parabens and develop rashes when using paraben-based moisturizers or anti-ageing creams. There are other preservatives which are safer than parabens and one can opt for these if the skin is allergic or sensitive to them.

9. Dermatologist-approved: This does not mean it is FDA-approved. The approval of any one dermatologist, who may even be working for the manufacturing company, is enough to label the product as 'dermatologist-approved'. So do not go by it.

10. Clinically tested: No doubt most of the branded products undergo a lot of research. However, there are no regulations as to how the trials are done. We don't know whether all the ingredients are tested or just one or two active ingredients. Consumers should not be misled by this term.

11. Organic: If 75–94 per cent ingredients in a product is organic, the product can be termed so, according to the US Department of Agriculture.

12. Natural: By calling a product natural, the manufacturer may mean that the active ingredients

are obtained from plants. But the product can still contain chemicals and preservatives to sustain it. Think about it, how can you use a papaya extract for days without it decaying? Home-made or freshly prepared products from extracts of a fruit or plant can be termed natural. However, they cannot be used for more than three or four days, even if refrigerated.

For basic selection, stick to the following rule:

Skin type	Label to look for
Oily or acne-prone skin	Non-comedogenic, oil-free
Dry skin	Hypoallergenic, should not be oil-free
Sensitive skin	Hypoallergenic, paraben-free, soap-free, fragrance-free

An excited Mickey said she would not only look out for the right labels for herself but educate her sister too. Her father, she said, would be the happiest because her sister would then not be wasting money any more.

WEEK 2

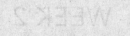
WEEK 2

5

Twenty Skin Myths

'If you fuel your journey on the opinion of others,
you are going to run out of gas'
—Dr Steve Maraboli

During our first meeting, Mickey emphasized on natural products only. She had never used anything on her skin before and so she didn't want anything with chemicals, especially before her wedding. All-natural wouldn't work in such a short span of time. There are many popular beliefs and myths regarding skincare. They may have been told to you by your grandmother when you were a teenager, or friends who subscribe to many blogs on the Internet, or those who gather at kitties and discuss skincare. Although they may all have been well meaning, there is no scientific evidence to that side of the story. Some of those advices are proverbial old wives' tales, others courtesy of Dr Google. Let us bust some of these myths.

1. *All-natural products are better for the skin.*

Natural is the 'in' thing. The question is: are the products really natural? Can you keep fresh orange juice in the refrigerator for over a week? It will decay, won't it? In order to keep natural things well preserved, preservatives are required. And preservatives are chemicals too. Quite often natural ingredients can cause irritation and allergies. I have seen reactions to some of the most common ingredients such as aloe vera and tea tree oil in people with sensitive skin. Firstly, the plants and trees whose leaves, bark or fruits are used should not be chemically treated or infused with pesticides. The soil in which they are grown should be organic too. Thirdly, the extracts must be pure. Then, the preservatives must also be natural. So always check the authenticity of the product and the manufacturer and do not forget to check the ingredients.

2. *You'll eventually outgrow acne.*

It is a popular belief that acne is a normal teenage problem. This is not true at all. Acne occurs due to hormonal changes in the body, especially when your androgen hormones increase. There can be many triggers for acne, such as stress, oil-based cosmetics, etc. (refer to the next chapter on acne for more details) irrespective of age. Acne can occur right from the teens to even the sixties. Adult acne is on the rise and just because you have never had a pimple during your teens does not mean you cannot have a pimple when you grow older.

3. *Expensive cosmetics are better than inexpensive ones.*

This is not true at all. A basic 30 g retinol cream which costs Rs 150 is as good as its branded equivalent which costs Rs 6500. Similarly, a basic cold cream is as good a face moisturizer, and Boroline a better lip cream than most of the fancy lip balms. Do not get lured by the packaging and do not be a victim of the fancy-looking skincare boutique. What is important is to look at the ingredients (common important ingredients have been mentioned in detail in chapter 3 and chapter 11), the date of manufacturing and expiry, whether the company which manufactures the product is authentic enough and finally whether the product is suitable for your skin.

4. *Hot water open pores, ice closes pores.*

I am sorry, pores do not open or close like a tap on their own, nor are they temperature-sensitive. A pore is an opening of the duct which carries sebum from the sebaceous gland to the surface of the skin. When the sebaceous glands secrete more oil or sebum, the ducts enlarge, giving the impression of an enlarged pore. Elastin fibres which hold the duct in shape lose their elasticity due to sun exposure or ageing. This can also cause the pores to become larger. While some anti-ageing serums and creams containing retinoids or peptides help in firming the elastin fibres, fractional lasers or micro-needling may help a bit more. However, there is no 100 per cent solution to open pores.

5. *Blackheads need to be scrubbed away.*

When too much oil or sebum is secreted by the sebaceous glands, the channels which take oil from the gland to the skin's surface get blocked just like a jam due to excess traffic. When this clogged oil, mixed with dead skin, reaches the surface of the skin, it gets oxidized and becomes a blackhead. It isn't dirt at all, so you cannot scrub it away completely. All you can manage to do is remove the upper part of the blackhead, and so it returns very soon. You need to use a salicylic acid– or lactic acid–based lotion or facewash which will exfoliate the lining of the pore and dissolve the oil, thus removing it completely. Scrubbing vigorously will only disrupt the protective layer of the skin, giving way to more microorganisms to enter the skin and cause more havoc.

6. *Drinking a lot of water will prevent acne* or *dryness and make the skin radiant.*

I often have these troubled patients who guzzle tonnes of water and yet have dry skin or acne. They are so distraught that water isn't doing the trick for them while it does wonders to people on the Internet. The good part about water is that it is extremely essential for our body to function well and remain hydrated. So we do need six to eight glasses of water a day. But water plays a small role in acne and dryness. It is the oil inside your skin, produced by the sebaceous glands (endogenous), and outside, in the form of moisturizers (exogenous), which is responsible for how dry or oily your skin actually is. So if your skin is dry, make sure to use moisturizers rather than simply drinking four litres of water a day. And if you have acne or oily skin, use products to reduce the oil or get to the root cause and treat it. Do not expect water to be a miracle worker. Our liver does all the detoxing and the digestive system or the urinary system flushes out the toxins. Water certainly aids them to function better. So drink water for their sake.

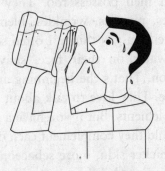

Drinking gallons of water

7. *Any cream or serum if applied for long stops working because the skin gets used to it.*

'Doc, the serum you prescribed was fab the first two months and then it stopped working,' is something I often hear from my patients. The truth is, your skin has its requirements depending on the climate, the environment, your hormones, the products you put together for your skin ritual. So how will a cream which was amazing in summer, when you were sweating most of the time, work in winter when your skin is cracking up? Don't forget that your skin is an organ; it will change with time and age. So you do need to change products. You may go back to the ones you have used in the past, depending on the skin condition.

8. *Skincare is a girl thing.*

I wonder why so many people believe this. Skin is something that men possess too. They can also have eczemas, rashes, pimples, wrinkles, blemishes. So why should skincare be a girl thing? I often see my brothers splash some water on their face, shave and use an aftershave lotion. That's the beginning and end of their skincare regime. They love to talk about fitness, protein and other supplements. But if you have a good body and a dull face, would they complement each other? Yes, men have slightly thicker skin, more sebaceous glands, more collagen. So they need different products. Men needn't keep a bunch of flowery or pink products which exude sweet fragrance in the bathroom or on the dressing table. I tell my husband to do me a favour by just using a sunscreen in the day and a moisturizer at night. Even this is more than enough. And if you follow the entire skincare ritual, you will surely have radiant, blemish-free skin.

9. *I will grow hair like a gorilla if I shave my hair.*

When you shave, you snip hair from the skin's surface. The hair follicle is not plucked from its root. So what

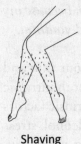

Shaving

you see are blunt edges of the hair when your hair begins to grow after a shave. These blunt edges give you an illusion of thicker hair but the reality is: there is no difference in the density or diameter of the strand. Imagine chopping the stem of a plant halfway—won't you find a rough edge? If you remove the entire plant from its roots, the surface of the earth is smooth. That's the case with hair too. When you wax, you remove hair from its root. So it regrows at a slower pace and the tapered ends of the hair are thinner, and the hair appears to grow thinner.

10. *If I pluck one white hair, I will grow many strands of white hair back.*

I wish that were true—I would pluck the few strands of grey hair from my brother Nikhil's scalp, so they would grow back in larger numbers! At least then he wouldn't bother about his receding hairline. White or grey hair is a result of the loss of a pigment called melanin in the hair roots and the skin around it. So if you pluck one grey hair, the new hair which grows will grow back white or grey because the melanin-producing cells in the hair root and its surrounding area have died. Which is why, sometimes, more hair which grow from this portion of the scalp will all grow white or grey. Remember that frequent plucking will damage the follicle, and hair may not grow back at all. You may even develop scarring and infection. So it's best to refrain from plucking your hair.

11. *I won't develop wrinkles or pigmentation because my mom's skin at sixty is still so radiant and youthful.*

It's true that genes play a big role in how your skin and facial features are. But ageing is based on both intrinsic and extrinsic factors. Your genes are the intrinsic factors but sun exposure, poor lifestyle, smoking, alcohol, stress and pollution play a huge role in shaping your skin, especially after you cross the forty mark. No matter how good your mom's skin is at sixty, you could still look like you are fifty at forty if you don't take care of your skin. Sun protection, healthy food, exercise, beauty sleep and no addictive habits are the key to good skin even in later years. Of course, you will need a little support from dermatologists in the form of a fruit peel or a non-surgical skin tightening once you cross forty-five or fifty.

12. *Regular facials are a must once I turn thirty to prevent ageing.*

Amid the humdrum of daily routine and busy schedules, facials can be stress-relieving and have a relaxing effect. The radiance on the face is a result of thorough cleansing but it's at best temporary and can also be achieved at home. Facial massages have a calming effect, but science has proved that massages neither improve circulation nor cause any lymphatic drainage. A study done in University of Wisconsin-Stout, USA, showed that massage therapy's effect on the stress hormone called cortisol is 'generally very small and, in most cases, not statistically distinguishable from zero' as opposed to the claims that massages can reduce cortisol levels.[*]

Secondly, nothing can be massaged into the skin to the point that it reaches the liver and detoxes it. This is more voodoo than truth. Applying things that enter blood circulation would be considered drugs and would have to be regulated by the FDA. Also fluid build-up on the face cannot be reduced by facials. That is a function of the kidneys. Sun protection is the single most important thing to ensure your skin looks good for a long time. Facials are a feel-good factor. Neither are they a compulsion nor do they stimulate collagen or tighten your skin or cause any lymphatic drainage or body detox. I do not discourage facials because it is nice to relax once in a while and have your skin cleansed too.

13. *I sleep well but I have dark circles.*

Yes, inadequate sleep is hugely responsible for the dark circles under your eyes but there are various other reasons too. Low haemoglobin, allergy to cosmetics or creams, dust allergies resulting in constant rubbing of eyes, asthma, hay fever, genes and certain medication can also cause dark circles in spite of you having your eight hours of beauty sleep every day. So try to find out the cause and get it treated accordingly. Your dark circles will certainly reduce.

---

[*] C.A. Moyer et al, 'Does Massage Therapy Reduce Cortisol? A Comprehensive Quantitative Review', *Journal of Bodywork and Movement Therapies* 1 (15 January 2011): 3–14.

14. *Oiling the hair is important for hair growth.*

When I look at all my childhood pictures, I wonder what my mom and my granny thought as they oiled my hair. I never really ended up with Rapunzel's hair but I surely looked like this nerd with oily hair tied up in a ponytail. Oil is a very good conditioner for hair. It helps reduce frizz and nourishes the hair shaft. However, coconut oil, almond oil or mustard oil will stimulate the hair follicles to grow new hair or make the hair shaft thicker. Some of the newer oils claim to have medicinal benefits but they have no scientific data to back them up. Oiling your hair (not the scalp), once a week for about two hours before shampoo, conditions it well and is a healthy hair practice as long as you are clear that it will neither stop your hair fall nor promote hair growth.

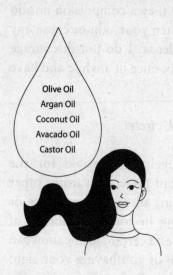

Olive Oil
Argan Oil
Coconut Oil
Avacado Oil
Castor Oil

15. *I will develop wrinkles if I do not apply moisturizer and foundation in upward strokes.*

This is completely untrue. You cannot rub wrinkles into your face, nor can you alter your muscles or fat just by using your make-up in upward strokes. In young people, the skin is more elastic. So when you stretch it, it bounces back. In mature skin, the elastin fibres are weaker and the skin is not so supple due to the loss of elasticity. So when you sleep with the same side of your face squished into the pillow every day, you will develop more wrinkles and sagging on that side of the face. Instead of focusing on the movement of your hands while applying make-up, train your mind to sleep straight on your back rather than curling up on one side.

16. *I will be able to get rid of my wrinkles with facial exercises.*

Exercise does help to tone your body and is extremely good for your skin and overall health. But facial exercises have to be taken with a pinch of salt. Constant movement of muscles will cause more lines and wrinkles rather than reducing them. Actors and people who emote more as they speak always end up with more wrinkles. A report in the *Aesthetic Surgery Journal* published in 2014 showed that facial exercises do not play a role in facial rejuvenation. Hence it is better to stick to squats in the gym than exercising your face in front of your dressing mirror.[*]

---

[*] Van Borsel et al., 'The Effectiveness of Facial Exercises for Facial Rejuvenation: A Systematic Review', *Aesthetic Surgery Journal* 34, no. 1 (1 January 2014): 22–27.

17. *Toothpaste is the quick fix to my pimple.*

Most teenagers who consult me for their acne have already tried dabbing toothpaste on their pimple in the hope that it will disappear. This is an old hack which won't work now. The older formulations of toothpaste contained an ingredient called triclosan, which killed acne-causing bacteria. So it did help to dab toothpaste on your acne. However, triclosan was found to reduce the immunity in children who were exposed to antibacterials at an early age. Hence, newer toothpastes stopped including it as an ingredient. As a matter of fact, some of the current ingredients may lead to irritation and rashes. So stop applying toothpaste on your pimple a day before your prom night. You don't want a rash on your face which you can't even conceal with make-up.

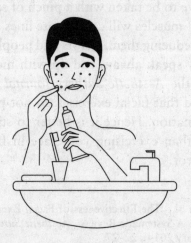

Toothpaste on a zit

18. *Wine and dark chocolate are great for the skin.*

While red wine has resveratrol, a powerful antioxidant, having it every day in the name of beauty can actually be detrimental to your skin. It can leave your skin dehydrated, sallow and wrinkled. You could also end up with puffy eyes. A glass of red wine once in a while is good enough. You might as well gorge on cranberries, blueberries, dark grapes, pistachios and peanuts to get your resveratrol.

Dark chocolate has cacao which contains resveratrol and polyphenol antioxidants. But you should look for 80 per cent dark chocolate with minimum sugar if you want to actually benefit from it. You can't have any chocolate considering it to be good for your skin. On the contrary, sugar causes glycation, which results in early signs of ageing.

19. *I will become fair if I take glutathione injections.*

Glutathione is a powerful antioxidant used for the treatment of liver disorders. It can be taken in the form of tablets or aerosol sprays for its antioxidant benefits. The dose is 600–1200 mg/day and not more. Skin lightening is a side effect of glutathione, as it depletes the pigment melanin from the skin. However, not everybody develops a side effect. Moreover, for the side effect to persist, you will need to continue taking glutathione. Once you stop it, your colour may go back to what it used to be within a year or so, sometimes even earlier. And if you do not develop a side effect to glutathione, it will not make your skin lighter unless you overdose yourself. It is not yet US FDA approved.

20. *A body detox will keep my skin allergies and pimples away.*

We abuse our body day in and day out with unhealthy food, stress, pollution, sun exposure, poor sleep, sedentary lifestyle and so on. It is good to give the body some rest and take a break from all the abuse. You can detox your body by living on greens and natural food, drinking a lot of water and taking ample rest. This is easy on the gut and helps clear a lot of waste which accumulates in our intestines for days. It is also good for the liver and intestines; however, it will not have much of an effect on your hormones or on the immune system of your body. Hence you may still break out into acne or develop a rash as there is no correlation between detox and the skin.

'Oh my God, doc! You've busted so many myths that were stuck in my head too. Incomplete knowledge is so dangerous,' Mickey exclaimed.

There are a lot of myths when it comes to skin and beauty. No doubt the Internet is a well of knowledge but one must only trust authentic websites and articles written by qualified doctors when it comes to skin.

6

Acne

'It is not only for what we do that we are held
responsible, but also for what we do not do'
                                        —Molière

'I don't get pimples or acne, doc. But blackheads take no
time to find a lace on my nose. No amount of nose strips
help,' Mickey complained. Well, Mickey, blackheads
are a form of acne too. Let me give you a little insight
into acne.

One of the most distressing things that can happen
to you is an eruption of an unsightly pimple on your face
right before your birthday party or before that important
presentation you have to make.

In my eighteen years of practice, I have seen how acne
can have a depressing psychological impact on people. If
we doctors help these youngsters get rid of their acne, we
actually help them gain confidence and start a new life.

Take the case of twenty-seven-year-old Maitri who
was brought to my clinic by her parents. At her age if her

parents have had to bring her to a skin clinic, something must be surely amiss. I soon learnt that Maitri has been suffering from acne since the age of fifteen and was always disturbed about it. Initially her parents thought it was normal, so they did not take her to a doctor. After a couple of years, Maitri went to beauty parlours to seek help. She even applied home-made packs her friends and relatives suggested. She started eating healthy, chewed neem leaves and had *dudhi* (green gourd) in every meal since she had read on the Internet that these help in combating acne.

When nothing helped, she started to withdraw into a shell of her own. Worried, her parents took her to their family doctor, who prescribed anti-acne medicines. Maitri started improving, to her parents' delight. But as soon as she stopped the medicines, the acne came back. Her parents then took her for alternative therapies since allopathy wasn't working for their daughter.

By then, Maitri had developed big pimples, deep pits and dark blemishes, leaving her devastated. She did not want to meet anyone. She didn't go to college. She had become a complete recluse. She wasn't willing to get married because she was embarrassed to show her face in public. I got Maitri investigated for PCOS, and, as I had suspected, it was positive. I sent her to a gynaecologist to get the PCOS treated. Simultaneously, I started her on anti-acne treatments. Her acne settled completely within four months. Then I began my combination of chemical peels and fractional laser. In another six months, her scars had reduced by 70 per cent.

One day, almost after a year of treatment, Maitri walked into my clinic with a cake and a huge smile on her face. She was dressed well, had lipstick on (I had never seen her wear make-up before) and exuded a kind of confidence I had never seen in her. The cake was for two reasons, she said. First, it was her birthday. Second, her marriage was fixed and she would be married within three months. Today, Maitri is happily married and has a twelve-year-old kid, and I am her child's dermatologist too. And guess what her child comes to me for? Treatment of acne. Maitri says she doesn't want her daughter to go through the same mental trauma that she had undergone due to her problem. My profession certainly gives me a lot of gratification and joy and I thank God for this every day.

Acne is estimated to affect 9.4 per cent of the global population, making it the eighth-most prevalent disease worldwide.[*]

According to the Global Burden of Disease (GBD) study conducted in Seattle University, Washington, in 2013, acne vulgaris affects 85 per cent of young adults aged twelve to twenty-five. Acne persists into the twenties in around 64 per cent of individuals and into thirties in 43 per cent of individuals. It is seen that 15–20 per cent females in their forties and fifties suffer from acne and 7–12 per cent of males have acne in their forties and fifties.

In my own practice, I see about forty to fifty patients a day and almost 40 per cent of them suffer from acne.

But first we need to understand what the difference between pimples and acne is. I often have youngsters

---

[*] J.K. Tan and Ketaki Bhate, 'A Global Perspective on the Epidemiology of Acne', *British Journal of Dermatology* 172 (July 2015): 3–12.

come to me and say, 'I don't get pimples or acne but I do get blackheads and whiteheads. So I keep scrubbing my face to get rid of them. But they keep popping up again and again.'

Let's clear this common confusion in our minds. Acne is a medical term for blackheads, whiteheads, pimples, pustules, cysts, nodules (pimples that don't come out on the surface but just seem like hard bumps inside the skin).

If you have blackheads and whiteheads, in medical terms it will be called grade 1 acne. This is the mildest form of acne. If you have tiny pus-filled pimples, they are grade 2 acne. Grade 2 is a more severe variety of acne. Large, painful pimples, some of which look like cysts, are grade 3 acne. This is obviously more severe than grade 2 and will need stronger medicines for a longer duration. And if you have a mix of all of these and those red bumps which never come out, you have grade 4 acne. This is the most severe form and usually there is a severe hormonal issue in such cases.

Now that this has been clarified, let's talk about who can get acne. My friend Mehek, who is my age, came raging to me one day and said, 'Why am I suddenly getting pimples? *Jawani ab kyon aa rahi hai*, I never had them in my teens!'

Well, my dear friend, there is no age for this notorious thing called acne. Yes, they are more common during teenage because of the natural process of puberty and hormonal changes in the body—you have heard that a million times—and it's androgens, or the 'male' hormones, that are responsible.

Male hormones in females? I am not kidding. Females have a bit of male hormones and males have a bit of female hormones for proper functioning of the human machine. These hormones never leave us. When women get pregnant, or are heading towards menopause, their hormones go haywire. Irrespective of our sex, when we are stressed, our hormones go haywire. So when androgens increase—whether in males or females—pimples can occur even in the thirties and forties.

Why does this happen?

As I mentioned, the most common cause of acne is a hormonal imbalance in the body. It could be a natural result of teenage both in males and in females. In females it can also occur before menstruation, during pregnancy or before menopause or as a part of PCOS.

Stress is the second most common cause. Stress causes an increase in cortisol levels. This sends signals to our brain and the brain then gives signals to the oil glands to secrete more oil and result in acne.

Another reason for acne could be the intake of drugs such as steroids, body-building supplements and other hormones.

Acne can also appear if your pores get blocked due to application of creams and lotions which have an oil base. These creams and lotions are easy to identify as they leave a layer of moisture on the skin's surface and are greasy to the touch. Also, upon sweating due to exercise or running, the water in the sweat evaporates, leaving behind sweat salts on the skin which could also block the pores.

When our pores get clogged, the natural oils cannot flow out through the normal pores. They collect in the oil glands as a white cheesy substance called sebum. Now the normal bacteria called *Propionibacterium acnes* feed on sebum and multiply. Just like human population, anything in large numbers is bad, isn't it? So, the quiet and peaceful *Propionibacterium acnes* become notorious after having fed themselves well and are ready to attack the skin.

That's when pimples form.

Did you know that pollution and humidity have a huge role to play in the formation of pimples too? Studies have shown that presence of particulate matter from vehicles and industries can cause acne.[*]

And finally, the million-dollar question:

What about junk food?

There is research documenting that dairy as well as food with high glycaemic index have a role in acne. So those of you who suffer from pimples and zits and want to get rid of them have to divorce those chocolates, ice creams, milk shakes, smoothies, cheese, pizzas, burgers, cakes, pastries, potato chips and the like.

---

[*] A.E. Nel et al., 'Enhancement of Allergic Inflammation by the Interaction between Diesel Exhaust Particles and the Immune System', *Journal of Allergy and Clinical Immunology* 102 (1998): 539–54; J. Krutmann, et al., 'Pollution and Acne: Is There a Link?' *Clinical, Cosmetic an Investigational Dermatology* 10 (2017): 199–204.

Kucharska and others reviewed scientific literature and found that dairy and chocolate do aggravate acne.[*]

Acne is more common in people who are genetically pre-disposed, which means if your parents or grandparents suffered from acne, chances are you will have them too.

Why do people get acne on the shoulders and back?

Twenty-year-old Myrah's mom was traumatized by the fact that her daughter was getting these tiny eruptions all over her back. At the same time, thirty-two-year-old Anmol who was going to get married in a couple of months couldn't figure out why his chest was full of these ugly, painful boils. When I examined them and told them that they were suffering from acne, both had a similar reaction, 'Doc, how can acne occur on the chest and back?'

Acne can sprout on all the parts of the body which are rich in oil glands or sebaceous glands. While the face is the most common area, it can also erupt on the chest, back, shoulders, upper arms, buttocks and thighs.

Back, chest and shoulder acne are more common in people who work out and sweat more. They can also occur if you have dandruff. They are also more likely to occur if you take anabolic steroids or body-building growth hormones. It can even be a result of a very

---

[*] Alicja Kucharska, Agnieszka Szmurło and Beata Sińska, 'Significance of Diet in Treated and Untreated Acne Vulgaris', *Advances in Dermatology and Allergology* 33, no. 2 (2016): 81–86.

relaxing oil massage on the body. So next time you want an oil massage, you will have to think twice if you have had acne on the back anytime in the past.

Not just that. Your hair conditioner too can cause acne on the chest and back. Most conditioners contain oil-based ingredients such as jojoba oil, petroleum, shea butter or silicone which clog the pores and cause acne. After rinsing the conditioner off your scalp, use a shower gel to wash your chest and back thoroughly, making sure there is no residue of the hair conditioner left on your body. Also make sure you wash your face.

Aman had the issue of hairline acne. He was so fond of his hair gels and sprays that he was just not ready to part with them when I pointed out that they could be causing the hairline acne. Finally, I gave him a little tip. I asked him to look for hair products which did not contain myristyl myristate. Myristyl myristate used in hair products and isopropyl myristate in creams and lotions can cause acne and should be avoided if you have acne-prone skin or are suffering from it.

Should teenagers be taking medicines for acne?

Most parents come and complain that since their boys don't wash their faces often, eat all the wrong food and don't sleep on time, they get pimples. 'Doc, Virat is just seventeen, please don't prescribe medicines but just tell my son how to take care of his skin so that he doesn't get acne,' a mother said to me.

Parents, I completely agree with you on the fact that a proper skincare routine should be followed. But whether medicines be prescribed or not depends on the severity of the acne and the hormonal imbalance. If there are large cysts, they will leave scars on the face. In such cases, oral medication is necessary.

So all you buddies who have zits, pimples, blackheads, breakouts, acne—whatever you call them—let's begin with your skincare routine first.

Make sure you wash your face at least twice a day. If you have really oily skin, you need a facewash which has salicylic acid in it. Salicylic acid is obtained from willow birch trees. It is a beta hydroxy acid which unclogs the pores and reduces the oils. It also helps in gentle exfoliation of the dead skin. However, if you have acne and are using anti-acne creams which contain retinoids like tretinoin, adapalene or even benzoyl peroxide, or taking some oral medication like isotretinoin, you may have to think twice before using salicylic acid. These ingredients make your skin dry and flaky. Using salicylic acid on dry skin can increase the dryness and irritate the skin. In such cases what you need is a mild cleansing lotion which has no soap.

Never overdo the cleansing routine. Washing twice a day is more than enough. However, if you sweat due to exercise or after playing a sport, you will have to cleanse your face even if it's for the third time.

Over-cleansing is harmful to the skin. The protective barrier layer called the lipid bilayer as well as the skin's natural moisturizing factors get ripped off by washing too much or too frequently.

'What about clarisonic brushes and scrubs?' asked Mickey, amused with the idea of brushes for the face.

Clarisonic brushes are great if you have oily skin and a lot of acne. But don't use them every day. Scrubs and clarisonic brushes can be used once or twice a week if you have acne-prone skin.

What about multani mitti and home-made packs?

Multani mitti or fuller's earth can be mixed with water or rose water and applied on the face for ten minutes and rinsed. It dries the face and removes oil and grime. However, do it only once a week or else it will rip away the moisture from your skin.

Not everything that you read on the Internet is safe. Avoid using milk, yogurt, milk cream (malai), facial oils, limes, lemons, tomatoes or potatoes on your skin. Oils, milk and milk products can lead to more whiteheads, while tomatoes and lemon can irritate the already irritated skin.

So what can you use?

- Make a coarse powder of oats, add a spoonful of honey to it to make a paste and use this as a scrub.
- You can also use mashed papaya.
- A fine powder made out of masoor dal can be mixed with rose water and used as a scrub too.
- Finally, a paste of tulsi and neem leaves with a pinch of pure turmeric can be mixed with water and applied on the face for ten minutes.

Never leave any of the packs, however natural they may be, for more than ten to fifteen minutes.

Kiara has normal skin and her brother has oily skin. Take a guess. Kiara never forgets her skin toning ritual while her brother never bothers to use a toner. Which of them is doing the wrong thing?

Well, neither of them is wrong.

A toner cleanses deeper, unclogs pores and removes make-up. If you have normal or dry skin, you really do not need a toner. If you have oily skin, you could use a toner in addition to a cleanser especially if you use a lot of make-up. Avoid alcohol-based toners. Pure rose water can also be used as a toner instead of synthetic preparations.

Yamini thinks it is not important to use a moisturizer. She calls her face an oil factory because it secretes too much oil.

Yamini is wrong. Even oily skin gets abused throughout the day because of exposure to UV rays, heat, dust, pollution and stress. It does need a little comfort in the form of an oil-free moisturizer. There are plenty of water-based, oil-free moisturizers available and should be used at least once a day. Whether you apply it during the day or night doesn't matter.

Kunal hates sunscreens. Sunscreen makes his face sticky and white, and he thinks it causes his acne problem to rise. I hate to say this but Kunal is wrong. When acne heals, they may leave behind their traces in the form of blemishes. These blemishes may stay for months together if you do not protect yourself from the harsh UVA rays. So you must use a sunscreen with SPF 30. There are gel-based sunscreens, or matte sunscreens which are neither greasy nor leave a white film on your skin. Pick any one of them and apply fifteen minutes before stepping out in the sun.

What about anti-acne creams?

If you have pus-filled yellow zits, you may use a clindamycin gel at bedtime. If you have blackheads or whiteheads, try 2.5 per cent benzoyl peroxide gel once a day. However, if your acne does not subside or if you develop large cysts or nodules, you must consult a dermatologist.

All females above eighteen years of age must do their blood hormone tests and ultrasound of the ovaries to rule out PCOS. These should be done between the second and the fifth day of the menstrual cycle for accurate results.

Krisha is an actor who needs to use cosmetics every day. She has grade 3 acne too. So I asked her to use an oil-free moisturizer with SPF, followed by a stick concealer instead of a cream-based one, and then a water-based, light foundation. She made sure all her cosmetics read non-comedogenic, meaning they don't cause comedones. However, be cautious, not every product which says 'non-comedogenic' really prevents acne.

Zubin has been banned from meeting me unless and until he stops picking at his acne. When you pick at or squeeze a pimple (I know it is very tempting), you actually damage the deeper layers of your skin, resulting in scarring and dark spots. These dark spots do not go away so easily. Days of creams and series of chemical peels are the only solution. Not only that, at any given point of time, we have thousands of germs on our skin, even if our hands are washed. When we squeeze a pimple, there is a direct gateway for these germs to enter the skin and cause more havoc. So please do not pick at your skin.

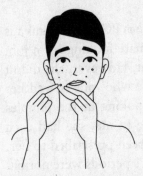

Popping a zit is a strict 'NO'

Britney had this strange problem. She would break out only on one side of the face. I inquired a little about her profession and lifestyle. She was a marketing executive and had to be on the phone every day. Her phone would be sticking to her right cheek whenever she used it. She had to travel quite a bit for her many meetings. And she would sleep on the right side of her face. She would break out into pimples on the right side of her face. Now this right-sided pimple puzzle was solved. Her cell phone could be carrying a lot of dust particles and microorganisms which can clog pores. The grime, soot and pollution due to her outdoor activities was only making her skin worse.

And finally, her maid would change pillow covers only every Sunday. Your face rests on the pillow for six to eight hours every night. So the pillow cover receives all the pore-clogging oils from your face as well as your skincare products if you haven't washed your face well before hitting the sack. This makes it a great breeding ground for bacteria. Your towels and face napkins can also harbour dirt and bacteria. I asked Britney to change her pillow covers every alternate day and use fresh face towels daily. I also advised her to clean her cell phone cover and keep it a little away from her face as she spoke, so that the phone did not touch her skin. In addition, I gave her a mild anti-acne cream, and magic happened. Her one-sided acne cleared up completely within five weeks.

Another common cause of acne is PCOS. Nayanika is a twenty-two-year-old MBA graduate looking for a job. She is tall, slim and very intelligent. However, she didn't have the confidence to face people who interviewed her because she felt they were only looking at the pimples on her face. By the time she came to me, she had used all the anti-acne creams that had been prescribed to her. But nothing had helped. Nayanika's periods were normal and I had little reason to suspect PCOS. Yet I decided to get her hormones checked. And guess what? Her reports showed raised androgen levels. An ultrasonography of the uterus and ovaries revealed multiple cysts in her ovaries. She is a classic case of lean PCOS. While 60 per cent females suffering from PCOS are obese or overweight, 40 per cent are actually lean and their diagnosis is often missed. Thirty per cent suffering from PCOS have normal periods.[*]

There is an explosion of PCOS in the last decade. When I had started my practice in the year 2000, I would see one patient with PCOS in three or four days. Now, one in every four females who walks into my consulting room has it. PCOS may be genetic or purely a lifestyle disorder. It presents itself differently in different individuals.

---

[*] Alicja Kucharska, Agnieszka Szmurło and Beata Sińska, 'Significance of Diet in Treated and Untreated Acne Vulgaris', *Advances in Dermatology and Allergology* 33, no. 2 (2016): 81–86.

According to a study conducted in 2011, prevalence of PCOS in Indian adolescent girls is 9.13 per cent.[*]

Some women suffer from PCOS without a hint until they find themselves struggling to get pregnant.

Approximately 40 per cent of patients with PCOS— both obese and lean—have insulin resistance. These women are at increased risk of type 2 diabetes mellitus and consequent cardiovascular complication. Insulin resistance is a condition in which the fat, muscle and liver cells do not respond properly to insulin and thus cannot absorb sugar from the blood. The body being an intelligent machine tries to produce more and more insulin to facilitate the absorption of glucose (sugar). This excess insulin sends signals to the ovaries to produce more testosterone, which is a male hormone. This leads to PCOS and even interferes with ovulatory cycles, leading to reproductive disorders. Ninety per cent of females suffering from PCOS have resistant or recurrent acne, 60 per cent have hirsutism (excessive hair growth on body), 20 per cent have acanthosis nigricans (thickened and dark skin folds) and 12.5 per cent have hair loss.

What about the cure?

While gynaecologists and endocrinologists prescribe certain medicines, lifestyle changes stand tall in the

---

[*] Nidhi R. et al., 'Prevalence of Polycystic Ovarian Syndrome in Indian Adolescents', *Journal of Pediatric and Adolescent Gynecology* 24, no. 4 (August 2011): 223–27.

treatment of PCOS. Eat right, exercise regularly, sleep on time, stress less, avoid alcohol and smoking and see the difference. Really tough in today's times of late-night parties, social media activity and WhatsApp chats at night! But if you want to have clear skin and suffer less, you have to lead a healthy lifestyle. There is no permanent cure for PCOS, but if you eat healthy and reduce weight such that your BMI drops to around 22–23, you will find your symptoms disappearing and your androgen levels going down to normal again.

High-fibre foods such as sprouts, beans, lentils, cauliflower, red leaf lettuce, bell peppers, broccoli, tomatoes, spinach, almonds, walnuts, olive oil, fruits such as blueberries and strawberries, and fatty fish high in omega-3 fatty acids, such as salmon, are great food options for those suffering from PCOS. Sugar, dairy and refined flour are a strict *no*.

So, my acne-prone friends, my honest advice to you is: Eat healthy, sleep early and for six hours, stay happy and stress-free. Meditate if you have to. Yoga helps too. This is your sure-shot way to clear skin.

Table 1

Labels to look for when you buy skincare products or cosmetics
Non-comedogenic
Oil-free
Water-based
Hypoallergenic
Matte

Table 2

Skincare product	Ingredient to look for	Ingredients to avoid	Examples of products
Face wash	Salicylic acid, glycolic acid, lactic acid	Sodium or ammonium lauryl sulfate	Sebamed clear foam face wash, Keracnyl face wash
Toner	Rose water, alcohol-free toner	SD Alcohol 40, denatured alcohol, ethanol and isopropyl alcohol	Rose water
Moisturizer	Aloe vera, glycolic acid, lactic acid, hyaluronic acid, jojoba oil	Mineral oil, petrolatum, isopropyl myristate and isopropyl palmitate	Sebamed clear face care gel, Acnemoist cream
Sunscreen	Zinc oxide, titanium dioxide, ecamsule, melanin	Benzophenones (like oxybenzone), cinnamates, octocrylene, certain preservatives like quaternium 15, and the fragrance Balsam of Peru	La shield lite, UV Smart, Suncros Tint
Night cream	Hyaluronic acid, retinol, benzoyl peroxide, vitamin C, Niacinamide, lactic acid, glycolic acid, salicylic acid	Shea butter, cocoa butter, coconut oil, lanolin, petrolatum, urea, borage oil	Yugard, Ega, Revibra C10
Make-up	Matte products	Thick or solid make-up products like stick or creamy compact foundations	

Mickey is confident she can deal with her blackheads now. She has realized that acne is indeed not just a hormonal but also a lifestyle disorder. The dermatologist can prescribe medicines, give you certain advice and do some treatments. Your acne will surely clear up but thereon remember, the ball lies in your court. Not only will you have to follow a proper skin ritual, you will also have to make certain lifestyle changes in order to see that you do not develop pimples all over again.

7

Hyperpigmentation

'When the clouds clear we shall know the colour of
the sky'

—Keorapetse Kgositsile

I met Mickey after almost ten days. She said she had been
religiously following my instructions. 'Doc, we forgot
my underarms. They are really dark,' she said at the
end. Dark underarms would need immediate attention
because even if you try to conceal dark skin with a
foundation, it will not stay when you get sweaty. And
Mickey had spent a bomb on her chic halter blouses to
match her saree and lehengas for the sangeet, mehendi
and wedding. Moreover, she was flying to the Maldives
for her honeymoon and would be wearing bikinis.
'Mickey, usually it takes about eight to ten months for
dark underarms to be fixed. But we do not have time.
So please get ready to undergo some laser treatments
ASAP.'

With this we started discussing pigmentation, a huge issue in India among both sexes.

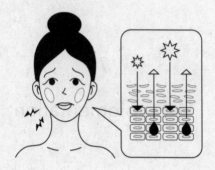

What is a pigmentary disorder?

Our skin has cells called melanocytes which contain a pigment called melanin. Melanin gives skin its colour. If there is increased melanin in a particular area of the skin, that area looks darker than the rest of the skin and is called hyperpigmentation. People also call them blemishes and dark patches on the face and body.

If there is less melanin in a particular part of the skin, that patch looks lighter and is called hypopigmentation.

Hyperpigmentation is a very common problem faced by millions of Indians. We have type 3 to type 5 skin, which means we always tan, never burn. This has its good side and bad side. The good side is that the melanin in our skin acts like a warrior protecting us from the harsh UV rays and preventing our skin from developing deep wrinkles or skin cancer. The ugly side, however, is that we tan easily and are prone to increased pigmentation.

Common types of hyperpigmentation

Dark underarms

The skin over our axillae (underarms) can get dark due to several reasons. It could occur as a result of a fungal infection which leaves behind dark patches. Another very common reason is allergy to deodorants and perfumes. Mickey literally pounced on me when I told her this. You may not wear perfumes in your underarms, but you do spray on to your clothes, and perfume being an aerosol, does manage its way to the skin through the clothes. Constant friction and pull due to hair removal as well as allergy to the soap that you use can also cause darkening of the underarm skin. If the underarm skin is dark as well as thick, it could be acanthosis nigricans, which is seen in PCOS, diabetes, obesity, hypothyroidism, etc.

While Mickey complained of dark underarms, Harita said she was embarrassed to wear a bikini because her groin (skin between her thighs) and her butt are very dark. This again is a result of a fungal infection or allergy to soap or constant friction due to rubbing of thighs or due to sitting for long hours (more so if you are a little overweight).

Solution

If dark underarms have become a menace, you need to stop all deodorants and perfumes and opt for some antifungal powders instead. Opt for laser hair removal to prevent more friction-induced hyperpigmentation. Lose weight if you are obese or even plump. Switch to a soap-free shower gel for bathing. Consult a dermatologist to see if you have a fungal infection. Investigate for diabetes, PCOS, etc. Apply a pigment lightening cream containing kojic acid. Salicylic acid peels and Q-switched Nd Yag laser are good treatment options.

Dark circles

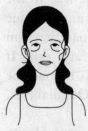

Dark circles

One day I happened to drop by my friend's place. She was busy trying to teach her twenty-one-year-old son how to use an orange corrector under the eyes. He had a prom night and he certainly didn't want to look like a raccoon with his prominent dark circles. Dark circles are a common concern—from teens to those in their seventies. Anyone can have them, no one loves to have them, but no one has been able to do anything about them. The most common cause of dark circles is lack of sleep. But there can be other reasons too. Low haemoglobin, smoking, poor lifestyle, excessive sun exposure or even liver disease can result in dark circles.

Rehmat has dark circles and so does her mother and grandmother. It runs in the family, she says. Yes, dark circles can be genetic too. Arjun is constantly sneezing and rubbing his eyes, as a result of which he has dark circles at the age of fifteen. Allergies to dust, pollen and even cosmetics can lead to itching and watering of eyes.

You must seek help from a doctor. Rubbing the eyes frequently will cause darkening of skin around the eyes. Your mascara, eyeliner, kohl, eye shadow and even your make-up remover could be possible culprits. Dark circles can also be a part of the ageing process. As one ages, the skin becomes thinner, there is loss of fat and blood vessels under the eyes become more prominent. They become sunken and hollow, casting a shadow under the eyes. This could sometimes be seen as tear trough in youngsters due to their bony formation from childhood.

Solution

First of all, bring discipline into your life. Stop scrolling through Instagram and Snapchat posts a million times to see how many likes you have got to the pic you posted in the evening. Avoid your late-night WhatsApp chats or watching your Amazon Prime videos. In fact, I would say, just switch off your cell phone at 10 p.m. Maybe 11 p.m. if I may be liberal. I do that every single day.

Sleep for a minimum of six hours every day. The eyes need rest and so does your skin. Quit smoking and drinking. Trust me, it isn't cool to be indulging in either. Alcohol can result in puffy eyes over time. So beware. Get your haemoglobin checked. If you have anaemia, make sure you take iron supplements and include food rich in iron such as spinach, okra, sweet potato, whole grains, brown rice, prunes, raisins, figs, fortified cereals, tofu and soybean in your diet.

Avoid rubbing your eyes and consult an allergy specialist if you suffer from allergies and sneezing.

Moisturize under your eyes at least twice a day and do not forget to apply a sunscreen too. Avoid cosmetics which could be responsible. At bedtime, clean your face, remove all make-up and gently dab an eye cream containing vitamin C, vitamin K and hyaluronic acid. If you suffer from severe dark circles, lactic and glycolic acid peels do help. You will need ten to twelve sessions at two-week intervals. If there is dark pigmentation under the eye, Q-switched Nd Yag laser treatment works best to get rid of the pigmentation or reduce it. I have explained more about this laser in chapter 18. Eyes should be protected while doing an under-eye laser treatment.

If you have sunken eyes and are above twenty-five years of age, you could consider getting a hyaluronic acid filler done. It is US FDA–approved, safe and lasts for a year, sometimes more. Never opt for permanent fillers in this area. (FDA gives approval for any medical product, be it medical equipment, lasers, injections, medicines or anything related to public health. The US FDA rules are extremely stringent and only safe, high-quality products receive approval.)

Dark patches on the cheeks

Every morning before leaving for work, Grishala closely inspects her face in the huge mirror on her bathroom wall. She comes back and does the same thing at night. Although she has no issues with her eyesight, she goes closer to the mirror and stretches her skin and looks on as if she would be able to gauge the depth of the dark patches on her cheeks. She has applied every possible cream and tried every home remedy that even the person sitting next to her in the train during her commute to work recommended, but her pigmentation only got darker, as if in revolt. As she looks in the mirror, she hopes that someday a genie would work his magic on her and when she wakes up, her cheeks would look rosy and radiant with no patches whatsoever.

There are millions like Grishala who suffer from a pigmentary disorder called melasma. This is seen most commonly on the cheeks and nose as if a butterfly has laid an imprint of its wings on the cheeks and its body on the nose of the face. It appears brownish in colour and may spread to the forehead, lower face as well as upper lip gradually. Grishala told me her melasma has a mind of its own. It increases on certain days and looks very light on certain days. Melasma looks darker just before one's menstrual cycle in females, or with the slightest of sun exposure or with stress. The latter is true in case of males too.

Melasma occurs as a result of sun exposure or due to hormonal changes in the body, for example, during pregnancy. It is very commonly seen in pregnant ladies and is often called the pregnancy mask. It can be genetic too.

Solution

Unfortunately there is no treatment which guarantees a permanent solution. Melasma will disappear if it is epidermal but may only lighten if the increased melanin is sitting deeper in the dermis. The most important treatment is protection from UVA, UVB rays, visible light and infrared rays. Use a broad-spectrum sunscreen, wear wide-brimmed hats, scarves, and carry an umbrella whenever possible. There are skin-lightening creams containing hydroquinone which form the gold standard. However, prolonged use of hydroquinone leads to blotchy skin and a condition called ochronosis. Tranexamic acid-based creams are found to be better and safer. They have no adverse effects even when used for a long period of time. We dermatologists also do microneedling with tranexamic acid and glycolic acid peels to lighten melasma. Some doctors like to use lasers to treat melasma but I personally refrain from it. I have seen in my practice that melasma always returns no matter how good the laser is.

Dark lips

I have always seen my neighbour Lavie wear bright red, maroon or orange lipsticks. Her latest favourite is violet. The dark colours look very sexy on her too. However, my son wondered why she wore lipstick at home too while I did not. I told him it was rude to say that and we should leave people to their choices and not have an opinion about everything. One day Lavie came to my clinic distressed. She removed her lipstick to unveil her dark, almost black lips. She was fed up of camouflaging them 24/7. Smoking is the most common cause of dark lips. Nicotine constricts the blood vessels, reducing the blood supply to your lips, causing them to dry and darken. Also tobacco is deposited on the lip mucosa and causes discoloration of the lips. Caffeine can have the same effect, which means too many cups of black tea and coffee can also be a reason.

Another very common cause of dark lips is lip licking. By pursing, biting or licking your lips constantly, you increase the chances of lip discoloration. Your own saliva becomes your enemy and damages your lip mucosa, making it dark and chapped.

An allergy to the silver coating on sweets and condiments or to colour in toothpastes, high content of lead in dark-coloured lipsticks, poor-quality lip balms, lip glosses and lipsticks can all result in the darkening of lips. Some drugs like amiodarone, daunorubicin, gold, methotrexate, psoralens and 5-fluorouracil given for autoimmune disorders can also cause the same effect.

Solution

First, stop smoking. Second, no more licking your lips or pursing even though they may feel dry as a bone. A lot of times, you lick your lips out of sheer habit, without even realizing it. You have to tell yourself time and again not to do so. That is the only way to train your subconscious mind and get out of the habit. Another solution is to carry a lip cream with you and keep applying it every two hours. Drink a lot of water so that you are not dehydrated. Avoid using dark shades of lipsticks and unknown brands. Avoid fragrance-based lip glosses and lip plumpers. Fragrance can induce pigmentation of lips. Use good old white-coloured toothpastes. Avoid having menthol and silver-coated sweets and condiments after your meal. Non-flavoured pure fennel seeds are good digestives instead of cloves and betel leaf.

Certain lip-lightening creams containing kojic acid, liquorice extract, niacinamide, arbutin, bearberry extract, mulberry extract, vitamin C and vitamin E help in reducing the lip colour.

Lactic and glycolic acid peels as well as Q-switched Nd Yag lasers are other options, albeit it takes many sessions and almost a year to get rid of the dark colour.

Dark patches on face (forehead or chin or entire face)

Thirty-five-year-old Vikrant has a dark patch on his forehead, almost like a band. On probing, he confessed to using a lot of balm during his teens as he suffered from migraines. Dark rough patches on the forehead and sides of the cheeks can also occur due to sun exposure, constant friction due to wiping of sweat or even in those who have insulin resistance or diabetes. Blotchy pigmentation can also be seen on the entire face and neck due to consumption of Ayurvedic *bhasma*s which contain heavy metal.

My cousin Rishabh came to me two months before his wedding wanting to get rid of his tan. His face, arms, hands and neck were four shades darker than the rest of the body. In fact, his chest and back looked like someone else's because they were so much fairer! Rishabh has a marketing job and travels most of the time. He has been doing this for eight years and before that he was a soccer player in school and college. Rishabh thought his skin was badly tanned. He was partially correct. When the skin is assaulted by repeated exposure to UV rays, the tan gets converted into hardcore deeper pigmentation. It doesn't remain the superficial tan which is supposed to regress on its own within three months of sun exposure. UV rays also increase freckles and cause sun spots.

Solution

Avoid sun exposure. I tell my patients they may forget to brush their teeth on a certain day but they should not forget to use a sunscreen 365 days of the year if they have any kind of pigmentation on any exposed part of the body.

Balms which claim to relieve headaches are counter-irritants. They contain menthol, camphor, peppermint, cajaput oil and clove oil which can irritate the skin and cause pigmentation. Stop using all balms if you have pigmentation or even the slightest family history of pigmentation.

Avoid wiping your sweat with thick Turkish napkins. Dab your face with dry tissues instead. Spray thermal water mist to wipe the sweat away. This will keep your skin cool and hydrated too.

A lot of powders, bhasmas and lotions claiming to be Ayurvedic contain heavy metals such as mercury and lead. Do not take them without consulting a qualified Ayurvedic physician. Hair colour or hair dyes have paraphenylenediamine (PPD) in them which is the key ingredient in dark colours such as black and brown. A lot of people may be allergic to PPD and they develop either blisters on the scalp, an itchy scalp, or pigmentation along the hairline which gradually spreads to the rest of the face. If you have such symptoms, you must use an organic hair colour or a vegetable dye. Henna is another option but it may leave a reddish tinge and even make the hair dry. So you will need to condition your hair well. Finally, foundations, essential oils and perfumes can cause or increase existing pigmentation. Avoid using them. Opt for a mineral powder if you have to use a foundation. Spray perfumes on to your clothes and wear them after ten minutes if you think you cannot do away with your perfumes.

Very importantly, you must consult a dermatologist. Firstly, because your skin may be trying to tell you something you do not know. These pigmented spots are like warning flags trying to tell you that you may be under attack. Hypothyroidism, diabetes, PCOS, hormonal imbalance, liver disorders, kidney disorders could all manifest with increased pigmentation in the beginning and should not be ignored. Secondly, your dermatologist will make a diagnosis and treat the cause rather than prescribing random skin-lightening creams which are available over the counter. Specific chemical peels and laser treatments can be performed to reduce or get rid of pigmentation, provided they are done by qualified dermatologists. Read chapter 18 to know more about these peel and laser treatments.

Dark neck

Twenty-year-old Sumaira yearns to wear noodle-strapped tops for parties like her friends do but ends up wearing turtleneck tops all the time because she is embarrassed to show her neck. The skin on her neck is thick, rough and dark. She keeps herself very clean but that really doesn't help. The thing to remember here is that the moment one says thick, dark, rough skin, a bell should ring—it could be insulin resistance, hypothyroidism, diabetes, PCOS, Cushing's disease or just obesity. This can happen on the neck, especially the nape. It can also be seen in underarms, groin and under the breast.

Solution

You must consult an endocrinologist and get your hormones checked. Work towards losing weight as well and stop rubbing your skin because friction will increase the pigmentation.

Dark elbows, knees and ankles

This occurs due to constant friction.

Solution

You must make a conscious effort to avoid sitting in a particular position which leads to friction of these parts of your body. Also make sure you always moisturize these areas at least twice a day. Keeping them hydrated will prevent friction and subsequent darkening of the skin. If they persist, you could opt for phenol and TCA peels. About six to eight sessions at three-week intervals will reduce the discolouration.

Dark patches on upper back and forearms

Apart from a sun tan, dark, mottled, pigmented spots appear most commonly on the forearms, upper back and shin due to months of UV exposure or friction or autoimmune conditions such as hypothyroidism and diabetes. This condition is called macular amyloidosis and is more common in females. The female to male ratio has been found to be 3:1. My friend Kiara, her mom and her aunt suffer from macular amyloidosis. Upon investigation, both her mom and aunt were found to have hypothyroidism. While Kiara was spared thyroid disorder, the culprit in her case was the loofah with which she used to scrub her back every day, not realizing that this was the cause of the hyperpigmentation.

Solution

Always wear a sunscreen with SPF 50 on all exposed parts. Never use nylon loofahs or scrubs. Wear full-sleeved clothes from sunrise to sunset. Get your thyroid hormones tested to rule out hypothyroidism. Also, do a blood test for glycosylated haemoglobin. This is a test to detect diabetes in its early stage. Salicylic acid and TCA peels have shown some improvement in this condition.

Dark spots on the skin after injury

Tatiana is always anal about the slightest scratch or boil on her body or even a small pimple on her face. 'Even if I don't touch them, they leave a dark mark,' she says. Some people have the tendency to hyperpigment with every little scratch, acne, injury or boil, or even with an allergic reaction. That is the tendency of their body. This is called post-inflammatory hyperpigmentation (PIH). PIH can also occur due to picking at the skin if there is a boil or acne or if the patient has got any skin treatment such as a chemical peel or microdermabrasion or laser done and stepped out in the sun immediately without using a sunscreen.

Also beware if a cream or lotion makes your skin look abnormally red. This could be a sign of skin irritation leading to a sure-shot PIH.

Solution

Always protect your skin from UV rays if you have got any skin treatments done. Use a broad-spectrum sunscreen liberally. Avoid picking at, scrubbing or peeling your skin.

As a child, I often saw my aunts slather their face with a skin-lightening cream. They probably thought they would get fair sooner if they applied loads of the cream. Do not apply more than a pea-size of any anti-ageing, pigment lightening or even anti-acne cream at a time on the face. If you see that your face has become red, consider it a warning signal. The only two products you can slather on your skin as much as you want are sunscreen and moisturizer. Consult a dermatologist to get your PIH sorted. Various pigment-lightening creams which are steroid-free are prescribed under supervision. There is an array of chemical peels available, such as glycolic acid, mandelic acid, arginine, kojic acid, lactic acid, salicylic acid, etc., for the treatment of PIH.

The seven sinisters

If you don't want to be plagued by hyperpigmentation, you must avoid the 7 Ss.

1. Sun exposure: Don't step out in the sun without wearing a sunscreen. Full-sleeved clothes, darker-coloured fabrics, wide-brimmed hats and scarves are also helpful.
2. Swimming: Avoid swimming, especially in outdoor pools. Chlorine and UV rays are a lethal combination for people who have pigmentation or for those who are prone to skin darkening or tan.
3. Smoking: Not only does nicotine constrict blood vessels and reduce blood circulation, it deposits free radicles in the skin and depletes the fighter

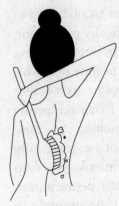

Scrubbing

antioxidants, resulting in darkening of skin and formation of wrinkles.

4. Scrubs: Do not scrub your skin vigorously or frequently. Much as it feels cleaner after scrubbing with fruit pits, nut fragments or polyethylene scrubbing beads, you could end up with increased pigmentation. Aggressive exfoliation damages the lipid layer of your skin, making it dry and prone to the detrimental effects of UV rays.

5. Stress: Stress can cause an increase in cortisol, leaving your skin vulnerable to pigmentation, acne and rashes. It is best to get into the zen mode. Keep calm and this will surely prevent increase in pigmentation.

6. Steam and sauna: Heat will rip the moisture off your skin and make it dry. Dry skin is more prone to damage from UV rays. Yes, it does feel relaxing to take steam or get into the sauna after a heavy workout but is it more precious than getting rid of your pigmentation? Think about it.

7. Scent: Allergies to any form of fragrance, be it perfumes, deodorants, fragrance used in preservatives, body talc, cosmetics, soaps, shampoos and even incense sticks, have been proven with research time and again. The most common way of allergy manifesting itself is through increased skin pigmentation. So you will have to give up all your lovely fragrance-based toiletries and cosmetics and make do with fragrance-free products.

Remember, hyperpigmentation can occur to anybody but is more common in those who are genetically prone to it. For example, you and your friend may both be pregnant but she may develop melasma while you may not. This does not mean you can bask in the sun for hours together without bothering about a sunscreen. Extrinsic factors such as sunlight, drugs, allergies and smoking can cause hyperpigmentation even if you may not be genetically prone to it. You must consult a dermatologist, who will identify the cause of your increased pigmentation or what's triggering it and then treat it accordingly in order to minimize or get rid of it. There is no single magic potion which would do the trick. But proper care and a committed holistic approach can make your skin look way better.

As for Mickey, I asked her to use an antifungal powder in the morning over her axillae to prevent any fungal infection from sweat. I also gave her a cream containing kojic acid and arbutin to use at night. I planned biweekly Q-switched Nd Yag laser treatments so that the pigmentation would reduce by at least 50–60 per cent. We still have five weeks to go. So am hoping to see some positive results.

8
Serums

'Everything has beauty, but not everyone sees it'
—Confucius

Mickey wanted to know if she should be using serums too. She was now gearing up to look her best on her big day. I usually prescribe serums to people as a part of their routine skincare after the age of thirty. But if people have dull skin or pigmentation, I do not hesitate to prescribe a vitamin C serum even if they are in their late teens or twenties.

When I was in my teens, I grew up watching my mom and aunts use Emami or Pond's cold cream every winter and Fair & Lovely or Vicco Turmeric almost like a ritual every night. Sunscreens became the next big thing when I turned twenty-one. When I entered my thirties, serums started doing the rounds. And now in my forties, I see the big hullabaloo about face oils.

What exactly is a serum? Just like the smartphone which has many functions and great power but is pocket-sized and light weight, serum is a lightweight, power-packed skincare product. A serum has highly concentrated formulations as opposed to a cream or a lotion. It is a more focused and target-oriented product, designed to cater to specific needs of the skin.

Serums have a fluid texture, they feel smooth on application and are much lighter than creams and lotions. They have a smaller molecular structure, due to which they can penetrate deeper into the skin, targeting specific skin needs at the cellular level. Serums can deliver higher concentrations of active ingredients such as vitamin C, peptides, etc. as they penetrate more easily into the skin due to their nanoparticle size. Secondly, serums are devoid of heavy moisturizing ingredients such as petrolatum, seed oil or mineral oil. Hence, they do not leave a thick layer on the skin. They are usually targeted towards issues like fine lines, pigmentation, open pores, blemishes and dull skin. They can even be incorporated in your routine skincare ritual to prevent fine lines, pigmentation and give your skin that extra sheen.

'Is it compulsory to use a serum?' asked Marissa who hates applying layers on her face and is always short of time. Well, cleansing, moisturizing and using a sunscreen are a compulsion as far as your skincare routine is concerned. Serums are for those who are looking to go that extra mile and want to have radiant, blemish-free skin.

'Are serums and face oils the same?' asked Samira, who got very confused when she went to a beauty store which showcased a plethora of products and the salesgirl tried to sell her almost every product, saying it was good for her skin. Yes and no! While traditional serums are water-based and are applied before applying a moisturizer, face oils are thicker molecules and they can replace a moisturizer. But if you have very dry skin, both serum and face oil may be needed. Face oils are marketed as oil-based serums too.

What about essence? Is it different from a serum? Actually, they are quite similar. Both need to be applied after cleansing, before moisturizing. Both are meant for targeted treatments. Both have microsized particles and penetrate deeper into the skin. But serums are a little gooey, while essences are more watery.

So to make it easier, if you have normal or combination skin, you can use a serum. If you have oily skin, opt for an essence. If you have dry skin, opt for an oil. Having said that, serums can go with all skin types but if you have sensitive skin, it is better to consult a dermatologist before splurging on a serum.

How do I know which serum is right for me?

Dry skin

Look for serums which contain hyaluronic acid, vitamin E, niacinamide, essential fatty acids, amino acids and ceramides. Hyaluronic acid is a natural moisturizer which keeps the skin supple and soft. Vitamin E is hydrating and is an antioxidant which protects the skin cells from oxidative damage. Niacinamide increases ceramide levels in the skin and prevents dryness. Lactic acid is a natural moisturizer. Essential fatty acids, ceramides and amino acids strengthen the skin's barrier layer and help build strong cell walls. They replenish naturally occurring skin lipids, aid in retaining moisture in the skin and protect the skin from pollution and environmental toxins.

Pigmented skin

Your serums should target the pigment cells and reduce the pigment. Glycolic acid, lactic acid, vitamin C and niacinamide are excellent ingredients when you have blemishes or a tan or pigmentation and you want to use a serum. Glycolic acid gently exfoliates and lightens the skin. Lactic acid is a mild skin-bleaching agent. Niacinamide or vitamin B3 has both hydrating and skin-lightening properties. Vitamin C fights environmental assault with its potent antioxidant properties. It also protects the skin from UV rays. In addition, it fights the bad enzyme tyrosinase, which is responsible for increasing pigmentation, thus preventing darkening of the skin.

Acne-prone or oily skin

You should look for retinol, salicylic acid, aloe vera or zinc-based serums. Salicylic acid unclogs pores; retinol reduces inflammation, kills germs and increases collagen production. It also helps in exfoliation and makes the skin luminous. Zinc regulates oil production and soothes the skin. Aloe vera is an anti-inflammatory agent. It prevents zits from turning into big pimples, it soothes and heals the skin and hydrates it too. You must opt for water-based, non-greasy serums.

Ageing skin

Your best bet would be a serum containing peptides, resveratrol, ferulic acid, vitamin C and vitamin E. All these ingredients are powerful antioxidants. They promote cell repair and new collagen formation, thus making the skin radiant and youthful. Peptides are known to boost elastin and collagen formation and restore the firmness of the skin. Grape-seed extract and pomegranate extract are also fabulous antioxidants which fight against free radicals and prevent fine lines from forming.

Where does a serum fit in my CHP routine?

A serum comes immediately after cleansing. Apply a moisturizer over the serum and then top it with a sunscreen. You can even use a serum before going to bed. If you want to use any other cream, layer it over the serum.

Serums are heavily concentrated. So a little goes a long way. Take two or three drops of serum and pat it on your face with your fingertip. Then gently massage it into your skin. This will be enough for your entire face. Too much of anything is bad and if it is a concentrated product, then certainly too much will cause irritation. So always remember to use very little serum, and refrain from using it altogether if you suffer from chronic skin conditions like rosacea or eczema.

Indication	Ingredient	Examples
Skin-lightening serum	Vitamin C, niacinamide, liquorice	Flavo C by Auriga, Revibra C10 by Dr Reddy's, VC 15 by Cipla
Anti-ageing serum	Peptides, retinol, vitamin C, hyaluronic acid	Ureadin anti-wrinkle serum lift by Isdin, VCx serum by Cipla
Hydrating serum	Hyaluronic acid, glycerine	Hyaluronic Acid Intensifier by SkinCeuticals, Cutisera intensive skincare serum by Cipla
Serum for acne-prone skin	Retinol, salicylic acid	Revibra A15 by Dr Reddy's, VC 20 by Cipla

Serums feel light on the skin and are easier to use since they don't leave a thick film on the face. They can be doubled up as a moisturizing primer before make-up, and because they are enriched with vitamins, antioxidants and moisturizing agents, they are safe to use. So if you too are getting married soon like Mickey, do not hesitate to ask your dermatologist which serum to use. And all those who are already married, I am sure that by just reading the chapter, you would be able to pick the right serum for yourself.

WEEK 3

9

Exfoliation

'Simplicity is the ultimate sophistication'
—Leonardo da Vinci

Now we were into week three and Mickey wanted to know why I hadn't asked her to exfoliate. All her friends believed in using scrubs almost every day for a fresher-looking skin.

Let us find out if Mickey's friends were doing the right thing.

Our skin is constantly working, even while we rest. Old cells migrate to the skin's surface from the deeper parts of the skin as a part of the normal cell cycle, which is twenty-eight days long. These old cells are dead and are shed through a process called desquamation or natural exfoliation. Skin begins to function more sluggishly as one ages, resulting in the piling-up of dead cells on the skin's surface. When light falls on this surface, it gets absorbed instead of getting reflected. This results in dull and unhealthy-looking skin. Exfoliation becomes important here.

Exfoliation is the process of removing dead skin cells from the upper layer of your skin. Not every individual can exfoliate. It can be detrimental if you suffer from eczemas, atopic dermatitis, inflamed skin, psoriasis and even sensitive skin.

Exfoliation can be done at home or at a skin clinic. Dermatologists will exfoliate your skin either by microdermabrasion or chemical peeling.

At home, you can use mechanical or chemical exfoliation techniques. Chemical exfoliation is done using alpha and beta hydroxy acids that are available in the form of creams and lotions. These acids gently dissolve the dead cells, making the dead skin peel off. Mechanical exfoliation is the fun part. It is done using scrubs with fruit pits or beads, with tools such as sponges or loofahs, clarisonic brushes and even a pumice stone.

Always select an exfoliation method that suits your skin type.

If you have oily skin, use scrubs with fruits, plant extracts or non-plastic beads. Plastic beads were banned in July 2017 as they go down the drain and pollute larger water bodies, harming aquatic creatures.

Pomegranate seed powder, jojoba bead granules, apricot scrubs, oatmeal scrubs, papaya enzyme scrubs, rice and wax are gentle mechanical exfoliators that can be used once or twice a week on oily skin.

If you have dry skin, opt for a mild AHA exfoliating lotion such as lactic acid or mandelic acid. This will remove the flakes that prevent the proper absorption of a moisturizer. Avoid physical exfoliators.

If you suffer from acne, opt for chemical exfoliators like glycolic acid or salicylic acid. These not only remove the grime, but also break down the pore-clogging dead cells. Physical scrubs are too harsh and can also irritate the inflamed skin, causing more break-outs and redness.

If you have sensitive skin, consider using a cleansing milk or an alcohol-free, enzyme-rich cleansing lotion instead of exfoliating the skin. Do not use gritty scrubs as they can damage the lipid layer of your skin.

Some exotic scrubs consist of blueberry extract, along with cranberry and raspberry enzymes. All of these are powerful antioxidants. They help slough away the dead skin to reveal the brightness underneath.

Another scrub I found has chrysanthemum extract, caffeine, sage and rosemary extracts. These deep-cleanse and have a calming effect on the skin.

Avoid exfoliation if you are using retinol-based creams or anti-acne preparations that dry up the skin. Exfoliating while using these products can worsen dry skin or even cause break-outs.

Never overdo the exfoliation ritual. It can cause more harm than good. Sometimes you may even end up with blemishes or pigmentation due to over-scrubbing.

How do you use an exfoliator?

First cleanse your face, removing all the make-up, sweat and grime that may have formed a layer on your skin. Then pat the scrub on the entire face. Using gentle, circular strokes, exfoliate for about thirty seconds. Rinse your face with lukewarm water. If you have open cuts or wounds or if your skin is sunburnt, do not exfoliate till the skin has healed completely.

After exfoliating, always use a moisturizer on slightly damp skin to keep it hydrated.

If you have very oily skin, you can exfoliate twice a week.

Exfoliating once a week is enough for those with normal skin. If you have dry or sensitive skin, do not exfoliate more than once a month. Exfoliating strips the skin of its natural moisture and makes it more sensitive and prone to rashes. It can also throw your natural oil production off balance and overcompensate, leading to acne.

Always listen to your skin. If it burns or turns red easily, it is telling you that it has had enough and you should stop scrubbing.

After listening to my lecture on exfoliation, Mickey decided to go the natural way.

She decided to make her own scrubs from kitchen ingredients as described in chapter 14 and exfoliate once in two weeks. Mickey had little time and I also wanted to do a bunch of treatments for her. So exfoliating frequently wasn't a great idea.

My advice

Seek a dermatologist's opinion on whether you should exfoliate or not and the type of exfoliation to pursue.

10

The Make-up Removing Ritual

'The purpose of art is washing the dust of daily life
off our souls'
—Pablo Picasso

Mickey had appointed a fabulous make-up artist who
would make her look like a million bucks at her wedding.
But obviously, the make-up artist would not accompany
her to the post-wedding parties and on her honeymoon.
So I decided to conduct a tutorial on cosmetics and make-
up removal. Mickey was really excited as she loved to buy
cosmetics and stack them on her dressing table. But I am
sure that after this lesson, she would not just pile things, she
would make the most of them and use them till the last bit.

When you go to buy cosmetics, ask yourself these
questions:

- What is my skin type?
- Is the product suited for someone my age?

- Do I have any skin concerns, such as acne, pigmentation, fine lines or flaking skin?
- What is the temperature of the place where I am going to use these cosmetics?

Teens and twenties

These days, I see a lot of young girls wearing heavy make-up to college to hide their pimple marks. This can clog pores and make pimples worse. Too much make-up can cause tiny break-outs even in normal or dry skin types. For those with a family history of pigmentation, it is better to keep it simple as foundations and concealers can cause pigmentation as well.

If you are in your teens or twenties, colourful lip glosses, tinted moisturizers and tinted sunscreens are your best bet for daily wear. This is the age when your oil glands are functioning well and your skin is hydrated. However, this is also the age where your skin easily breaks out into zits. So for special occasions, opt for a non-oily, lightweight liquid foundation. This will give you a sheer, natural cover.

Cosmetics for mature skin

Once you cross thirty, your skin starts to mature. You should now look for anti-ageing ingredients in your make-up products. Look for antioxidants, like niacinamide and vitamin C, and moisturizers like ceramides, in your foundation. Peptides and vitamin E are also good for anti-ageing. If you have dry skin, you should opt for a mousse or a cream or oil-based foundation. This will make your skin look smoother and more even. Foundations with SPF are even better as they will protect you from UV rays as well.

Most anti-ageing ingredients degrade on exposure to light and air. So look for products that contain anti-ageing ingredients and not just those that are labelled 'anti-ageing'. After thirty, the skin becomes drier. It is best to use cream-based concealers or sticks. Rich, creamy blush-ons are good alternatives to powders.

Acne-prone skin

If you have acne-prone skin, look for a non-comedogenic foundation with salicylic acid. Another ingredient to look for is dimethicone. It does not dry the face or clog the pores. In fact, it smoothens the fine scales found around drying pimples. Matte-finish liquid foundations are also suitable options. They provide good coverage, do not clog pores, last longer and reduce unwanted shine on the face. Thick make-up products, like stick or creamy compact foundations, provide high coverage but also cause great damage to the skin. They can trigger new zits or exacerbate existing acne.

One day, a twenty-three-year-old walked into my cabin with what looked like clear skin. After I removed all her make-up, all I could see were big black spots all over her face. These were caused by squeezing blackheads and whiteheads. To hide them, she used a thick concealer stick. This clogged her pores, causing more zits.

If you have oily or acne-prone skin and hate stepping out with blemishes, use a liquid concealer. Creamy and stick concealers only magnify the appearance of the pores, increase whiteheads and add an oily shine to the face. Powder blushes and bronzers are better options than gels or creams. Gels and creams can pool in enlarged pores and make acne worse.

Sensitive skin

Power foundations, especially those with silicon, are best for those with sensitive skin. Powder or cream concealers are safe bets. Mica and bismuth oxychloride add a sheen to the face and are usually found in mineral make-up. However, these two ingredients can cause irritation and itching. They should be avoided by those with sensitive skin.

Do not use fragrance-based make-up. It feels refreshing but does more harm than good. Avoid make-up with ingredients such as SD or denatured alcohol. Alcohol-based make-up is particularly harmful for acne-prone and sensitive skin. Avoid waterproof make-up, particularly for the eyes.

Removing eye make-up requires extra cleansing that can further irritate the skin. Use eye pencils instead of liquids, gels or kohls. Dark blue and grey eye shadows have more irritating chemicals and are avoidable. Opt for beige, cream and light pink shades instead. The wisest thing to do is to check ingredients and select brands that have fewer than ten ingredients.

Primers

Primers form a perfect canvas for foundation or concealer to set evenly on. They also help your make-up last longer. Opt for primers with an SPF 30 sunscreen. Also look for antioxidants such as coffee seed extract, apple fruit extract, green tea, green algae and soothing agents such as aloe vera, chamomile, liquorice and bisabolol. A combination of these ingredients helps shield the skin from sun damage, pollution, free radicals and toxins in the environment. Steer clear of alcohol- and fragrance-based primers.

BB creams

BB stands for beauty balm. These are essentially lightweight tinted moisturizers, usually with SPF. Newer BB creams contain antioxidants too. They have a creamy texture and are better for people with normal or dry skin.

CC creams

CC stands for colour correcting. These creams are meant to address issues like sallowness and redness. They are good for people with acne or oily skin.

BB and CC creams are not must-haves. A BB cream can be used instead of a moisturizer and foundation. But it does not provide adequate sun protection because it does not have adequate concentrations of the sunscreen ingredients. Besides, no one applies half a teaspoonful of

BB cream on the face and neck, which is the required quantity for adequate sun protection.

Mineral make-up

Mineral has been the buzz word for the last couple of years. Since mineral cosmetics are solid powders, there are no oil- or water-soluble phases. This makes it possible to eliminate the emulsifier, the most irritating ingredient in cream or liquid facial foundations. Mineral cosmetics are fragrance-, paraben- and preservative-free, making them safe for sensitive skin. They soak up oil and give a natural finish. That is why they are good option for those with oily skin too.

Another advantage of mineral make-up is that it contains zinc, iron and titanium oxide. These provide some protection from UV rays. However, mineral make-up isn't all natural the way we are made to believe. Some products may have ingredients like bismuth oxychloride, a byproduct of lead and copper processing, that are not minerals. They can aggravate acne, irritate the skin and cause rashes. If you have sensitive skin, avoid mineral powders that contain bismuth oxychloride.

Lip cosmetics

Most of us opt for long-lasting, matte lip cosmetics because we do not want to reapply the lipstick. But lips have no pores or oil glands. Air conditioners, room heaters, low temperatures and our own saliva can dry the lips. So if you are going to wear lipstick to work, and your work entails sitting in the AC for twelve hours at a stretch, choose a moisturizing lipstick.

If you have chapped lips, opt for glossy lipsticks. Choose lighter colours. Darker shades have more chemicals in them and make the lips drier. Avoid flavoured and coloured lip balms. Opt for colourless, odourless ones instead.

Often when you are getting ready for a party, you reach for a smudge-proof lipstick. After all, who would want their lip colour to slide on to their wine glass or coffee mug? Having said that, smudge-proof lipsticks do not contain oils and certain emollients that hydrate the lips. Hence, it would be all right to wear them on special occasions, but not as a part of routine wear. And if you have dry or chapped lips, smudge-proof, long-lasting lipsticks should be a big no-no. Long-lasting lipstick contains bromo acid that interacts with the mucosa (the wet lining in the inner part of the lip) and stains the lips red. This allows the colour to last longer, but also causes the lips to dry.

Dry lips also occur with the two-part lipstick that has an automatic cylinder with a sponge-tipped brush. One end of the cylinder contains a clear, unpigmented or lightly pigmented lip gloss. The other end has a thin coloured liquid polymer that binds to the lips for long-lasting colour. This polymer can block UV rays and is great when you want sun protection for your lips. The flip side is that it can cause irritation and dryness. One way out is to top it up with a moisturizing lipstick that not only adds colour, but also prevents dryness.

Can wearing lipstick every day cause cancer? This is a question I often get from concerned mothers whose daughters refuse to leave the house without painting their lips red. A couple of years ago, there was a big buzz about lipsticks containing lead. This was thought to be carcinogenic and toxic to the body.

The red pigments in lipsticks do contain lead. But the amount of lead is too small to cause any harm to the lips, except for staining them. In 2010, Frontier Global Sciences, Inc., under a contract with the FDA, tested 400 lipsticks from different brands. They found that only two lipsticks—Pink Petal Colour Sensational by Maybelline L'Oréal USA and Volcanic Colour Riche by L'Oréal USA—contained 7.19 ppm of lead. The remaining 398 lipsticks had less than 2 ppm lead in them. You would have to eat thousands of tubes of lipsticks every year to get lead poisoning!

However, to prevent lips from staining or turning dark, you should avoid wearing dark red or maroon shades every day. And if you still fear lead poisoning, you can opt for products coloured with fruit and other natural pigments.

What about lip plumpers? Lip plumpers are becoming increasingly popular. However, their use should be restricted to very specific occasions. Most lip plumpers contain capsaicin, menthol, cinnamon, ginger, niacin and even chilli pepper. These ingredients increase the blood flow by dilating the blood vessels in the lips. This causes the lips to swell, creating the illusion of plumper lips for a few hours. This can dehydrate the skin and harm the lip mucosa in the long run. Frequent use or overuse can cause scaling, dryness and even cuts on the lips. If you really want to use lip plumpers, look for ingredients like hyaluronic acid, peptides, marine collagen and human growth factors.

Eye cosmetics

The skin around the eyes is the thinnest and there are almost no oil glands here. This is why, for most people, the skin around the eyes can be dry, itchy and sensitive. The skin under the eyes also ages the fastest due to the structural anatomy in this region and facial movements. It is imperative to use a moisturizer around the eyes before applying make-up. Avoid waterproof make-up on a regular basis. It may be difficult to remove, resulting in under-eye puffiness and irritation the next morning. Eyeliner, kohl and mascara have a greater chance of entering our eyes as we toss and turn in our sleep. It is therefore important to remove eye make-up before going to bed.

False lashes

They are made up of natural or synthetic hair. They come in various shapes, sizes and colours. You can fix them to your own lashes with the help of a special glue. Make sure the angle of your false lashes and real lashes is the same so that they look natural. To remove them, use an oil-free eye make-up remover to soften the glue and then gently slide the false lashes off. Be careful not to remove some of your normal lashes. Store them in a clean plastic container for reuse. Some of you may be allergic to the glue and could develop allergic contact dermatitis. Always do a patch test with the glue and never use it if you have any eye infection.

Eyelash extensions

Eyelash extensions are a gorgeous, albeit expensive, way to enhance your natural eyelashes without mascara or false lashes. The lash extensions are made up of natural or synthetic hair. Each one is fixed to our own eyelashes with surgical glue. Extensions must be done by professionally certified and trained aestheticians. Lash extensions can cause allergies, dry eyes, itchy and swollen eyelids and eye infections. So one has to be extremely careful about the hygiene of the place, the sterility of the lashes and the expertise of the aesthetician.

Tips

1. Always cleanse your face well before applying make-up.
2. Apply a moisturizer on your entire face, don't forget the skin around your eyes.
3. Use a good primer if you want your make-up to last longer.
4. Avoid holding your phone against your face. It is full of microorganisms that can cause zits or tiny eruptions.
5. Avoid touching your face throughout the day. Your hands are not the most sterile things on earth.

6. Carry blotting papers with you to dab off sweat or excess oil that can cause make-up to slip and dissipate on the face.
7. Do not use expired products.
8. You need to discard products from time to time, even if they happen to be your favourite. Pay attention to the expiry dates.

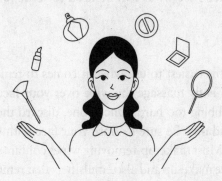

Make-up

Make-up product	How long you can keep once opened
Mascara and eyeliner	Three to six months
Cream, liquid or stick foundations and concealers, cream blushes	Six months to one year
Lip balm	One year
Lipstick, lip gloss and lip pencils	Two years
Powder-based products (e.g. blush, bronzer, highlighter, eye-shadow)	Two years

Make-up Removers

You are doing your skin a big favour by removing your make-up before going to bed. Not only do you allow your skin cells to repair themselves at night, you also wake up with glowing skin. Sleeping with make-up on can result in puffiness, rashes, itchy skin, milia and acne.

Now, let's see what can be used to remove make-up.

Wipes

Wipes are the easiest to use when it comes to removing light make-up. Gently massage the wipe over your face and eyes. Avoid scrubbing too hard. Once done, discard the wipe and use a second one. Be sure to rinse your face with water after doing this. Most make-up-removing wipes contain surfactants that dissolve make-up and also emulsifiers that remove oil, dirt and make-up. Hence the residue can be drying and irritating, particularly for those with sensitive or dry skin.

Avoid wipes that contain alcohol. They can cause a stinging sensation and dehydrate the skin. Opt for oil-based wipes, especially if you have dry or sensitive skin. They are gentle and usually free of phthalates, silicones, parabens and sulphates.

Micellar water

It isn't a fad. It is the real deal. Micellar water is almost like a water-based cleanser with barely any surfactants. It is made up of micelles, tiny balls of oil molecules suspended in soft water. These micelles attract oil and dirt and remove them without drying the skin. Micellar water is great for oily, acne-prone skin. They are usually alcohol-, paraben- and fragrance-free. So they are excellent for people with sensitive or flaky skin as well.

Cleansing lotion

If you have normal or dry skin and wear a lot of make-up, opt for a cleansing lotion. They do not contain soap or surfactants. They should be massaged gently on to the skin, left on for a few seconds and then wiped off with cotton pads. You may develop zits if you have oily or acne-prone skin.

Cleansing oil

You could use a cleansing oil from the beauty store, baby oil or even fresh almond or coconut oil from your kitchen. They all do the trick and remove highly resistant make-up such as glitter, bronzer and shimmer. But oils can seep into your pores and cause break-outs. So if you have oily skin, cleansing oils are not for you.

Eye make-up

Leaving eye make-up on overnight can result in eye infections, eye irritation, styes and broken eyelashes. A good eye make-up remover is one without alcohol, alpha hydroxyl acid and any kind of soaps or surfactants. Micellar waters remove eye make-up that is not layered or waterproof. But for waterproof or thick eye make-up, you may need baby oil or a special eye make-up remover. Baby oils do a great job at removing eye make-up. Soak a cotton pad in oil or make-up remover solution and gently press it down against your eye area. This helps the make-up to dissolve easily and reduces the amount of rubbing. Massage in a light, downward motion without pulling or tugging. You may end up pulling out your lashes or abrading the fragile skin around your eyes by rubbing too hard.

Tips

- Do not forget to remove every bit of your make-up before you hit the sack. You may have returned late from a party, wanting to crash immediately. But don't forget about your skin.
- I keep my cleansing pads by my bedside table. This always reminds me to remove my make-up before passing out.
- Soak a cotton pad in the make-up remover and then wipe the face gently. Allow it to sit on your skin for a few seconds in order to absorb all the make-up and grime. Now the make-up will come off easily without you having to scrub vigorously.
- Do not forget the eyebrows, eyelashes, lips, skin behind the ears, below the chin and the hairline.
- Do not rub hard to remove your make-up.
- Splash water on your face after removing your make-up. This will ensure no residue is left on your skin.

- Do not save on your make-up remover by trying to rub off all your make-up in one go. One cotton pad may not be enough. Use a second and a third one if required. Make sure you use a fresh side of the cotton or wipe every time you swipe. Otherwise you'll just redistribute the make-up particles.
- To kiss your long-lasting lipstick goodbye, spread a good amount of ghee or coconut oil all over your lips and leave it on for about fifteen seconds. Wipe this off with a cotton ball. The lipstick will come off without damaging the lip mucosa.
- Soak all your make-up brushes and sponges in a mug of soap water for at least half an hour every Sunday. Rinse them thoroughly. Make-up brushes, when not washed regularly, can collect microorganisms and dirt, leading to skin infections and allergic rashes.

Restoring your pH balance

Normal skin has an acidic pH of around 5 to 5.5. This pH is maintained by the acid mantle. It forms a protective barrier on the skin, blocking harmful bacteria, microorganisms and toxins, and restores moisture. Dry skin has alkaline pH, i.e. above 7. Hence it is more sensitive and prone to allergies and eczemas. pH-balanced products help restore the acid mantle and the protective lipid layer of the skin. They also help repair dry, flaky skin and skin wounds. Those with dry skin should avoid soaps and detergents as they make the skin more alkaline and increase dryness.

So now, when you wait in transit at various airports and end up visiting the lucrative cosmetic stores, make sure you buy the right stuff for yourself. And always remember, make-up isn't bad if you use the right products and, more importantly, remove it before going to bed.

Mickey has a lot of shopping to do and I am sure she is going to bless me for this tutorial. I hope you do too.

11

All about Anti-ageing

'What spirit is so empty and blind, that it cannot
recognize the fact that the foot is more noble than
the shoe, and skin more beautiful than the garment
with which it is clothed?'

—Michelangelo

One day a beautiful lady who seemed to be in her late forties
entered my clinic. She inquired about anti-ageing products.
In my clinic, when a patient comes in, they have to fill out a
form with details like name, age, address, etc. This lady had
left the age column blank. 'I want you to guess my age, doc,'
she said. After examining her, I said, 'Fifty?' I was close, she
was forty-eight. But she was devastated that I proclaimed her
to be two years older than she actually was. Although her
skin wasn't sagging and she didn't have wrinkles, this lady
had dilated pores and some fine lines. After going through
her skincare ritual, I added a few anti-ageing creams and
serums to her routine. At the end of the consultation, the
lady revealed she was none other than Mickey's mother.

Don't get worried by the term 'anti-ageing'. It's not always about Botox. Let us understand ageing before getting into age-defying products.

Anti-ageing means turning the clock back a few years. None of us can defy the process of ageing. But we can slow it down and age elegantly.

A young face is usually convex with full lips, a sweeping jaw line, full temples and cheeks. An aged face, on the other hand, is more concave with flat lips, sunken temples and cheeks, scalloped mandible and more shadows.

Ageing is a degenerative process caused by both intrinsic and extrinsic factors.

While the intrinsic or natural ageing process is genetically programmed and occurs evenly on all skin surfaces, superimposed changes at both the physical and the microscopic level occur because of environmental or extrinsic factors. These include sunlight, smoking, alcohol, weed, stress, pollution, irregular sleep, unhealthy diet and lack of exercise.

Intrinsic ageing normally begins in the mid-twenties. As a part of the physiological process, the cells in the lower part of the epidermis reach the surface within twenty-eight days in children and young adults. This cell renewal cycle slows down to forty to sixty days in those above the age of forty-five. What actually happens is, as we age, dead skin cells shed more slowly and there is a build-up of old cells on the skin's surface. The turnover of new skin cells decreases. This leads to dull, flaky skin. The moisture content in the skin reduces due to disruption in the protective lipid layer of the skin and reduction in hyaluronic acid content in the skin. Therefore, the skin becomes dry and dehydrated. The production of new collagen fibres slows down and older fibres shrivel up. The elastin fibres lose their spring too. Together, they result in loose, sagging skin and wrinkles in the form of furrows on your forehead, crow's feet, smile lines and turkey legs on the neck. Next to go as we age is the subcutaneous fat from under the eyes, temples, cheeks and even the chin. The bone and cartilage from the eye sockets, cheeks and nose is eaten up as well. Loss of fat and bone together results in hollow sockets under the eyes, hollow temples, hollow cheeks and a flat chin. Some of the fat gets redistributed to the lower face and leads to jowls, double chin and folds over the laugh lines. The nose begins to droop and so do the eyebrows and eyelids.

The signs of intrinsic ageing are fine wrinkles, thin and transparent skin, sagging skin, dry skin, inability to sweat sufficiently to cool the skin, greying hair, hair loss and unwanted hair.

Intrinsic ageing is responsible for 20 per cent of ageing changes. However, a whopping 80 per cent of the changes that we see in our skin as we age are due to extrinsic factors. So an anti-ageing regime involves a completely healthy lifestyle and a proper skincare routine.

When to start

Ritwik and Ayesha had just returned from their honeymoon. They completed their entire pre-marriage skin glow treatment package at my clinic and were now back with a new concern. They wanted their skin to continue looking radiant and not age! 'When should we start using anti-ageing products?' twenty-seven-year-old Ayesha asked. During the teens and twenties, the skin turnover is excellent and needs no extra support. The skin is capable of repair and can withstand the wear and tear.

What you need in your teens and twenties is protection and prevention. How do you do that? By using a broad-spectrum sunscreen. A broad-spectrum sunscreen is one that provides protection from both UVA and UVB rays. Occasional bursts of sun exposure while on vacation can be harmful. However, I believe that most sun damage occurs from daily sun exposure. Sometimes sun exposure is just incidental. You swear you are never in the sun but that daily walk from your car to the office door, the short trip to your terrace to dry clothes and the brief coffee break where you stare out of a glass window and watch the outside world are all enough to cause changes in your skin. The other important thing is to use is a good moisturizer, particularly at bedtime.

In your thirties, your skin is still doing well. It feels smooth and is pretty elastic. However, you suddenly notice that the skin tone is slightly uneven. A few fine lines may appear around the eyes. This is the decade where you should add vitamin C and retinoids to your skincare tool box. Vitamin C is a powerful antioxidant and prevents collagen degradation and pigmentation. Retinoids have been there forever. They are time-tested molecules that help speed up the cell turnover, build new collagen, reduce acne, shrink pores and even out the skin tone.

Retinoids, however, cause dryness and should be used in small quantities. Initially, use them on alternate nights. Then gradually incorporate them into your daily night routine. Retinoids should not be used by women who are planning to conceive or are pregnant or breastfeeding. They should also be stopped before a peel or laser treatment.

When you hit the forties, you need to focus on correction, along with protection and prevention. Pigmentation begins to set in in the form of melasma, freckles and pigmentary demarcation lines seen as dark patches on the sides of the cheeks. Fine lines become more prominent. You may see wrinkles in your mid or late forties even when you don't emote or talk. The oestrogen level drops around this time too and the skin starts to lose its radiance and firmness. The jowls and laugh lines become more noticeable. By the time you reach fifty, your neck and hands also begin to look wrinkled. Dryness sets in and sagging becomes a major issue. Now, along with your sunscreen, moisturizer, vitamin C serum and retinoid, you must use an anti-ageing cream too. Do not forget your eye cream and a cream for your neck and hands.

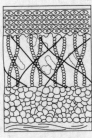
Skin at twenty

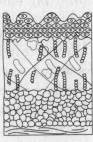
Skin at fifty

What to use

Just as the body needs a well-balanced diet, the skin needs a mixture of ingredients to maintain itself. A cleanser, sunscreen and moisturizer are must-haves. But once you turn thirty, you need to nourish the skin further.

Every skin type requires three categories of ingredients every day—skin-replenishing ingredients, skin-restoring ingredients and antioxidants.

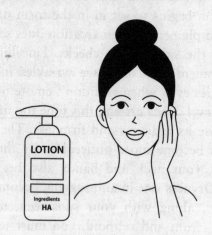

Ingredients

Skin-replenishing ingredients

These help moisturize the skin and revive the protective skin barrier. They fortify hydrating foods to the skin, making it smooth and supple.

Some of the skin-replenishing ingredients that you should look for in your moisturizers, day creams and night creams are hyaluronic acid, ceramides, fatty acids, cholesterol, glycerine, glycosaminoglycans, amino acids, sodium hyaluronate, sodium PCA, sphingolipids, glycolic acid and lactic acid.

Skin-restoring ingredients

These are ingredients found in most anti-ageing creams. They help tighten the existing collagen and elastin fibres, build new collagen, reduce unnecessary pigment in the different layers of the skin and improve skin roughness. Hence, they make the skin appear firm, youthful and blemish-free.

Skin-restoring ingredients are the anti-ageing superstar retinol, peptides, coenzyme Q10, resveratrol, grape seed extract, coffee berry, niacinamide, linoleic and linolenic acids, epigallocatechin-3-gallate (found in green tea) and adenosine.

Antioxidants

Free radicals are toxins in the body that can damage the DNA, proteins and lipids in the skin and cause cell damage. Our body is exposed to free radicals through pollution, soot, smoke, chemicals, digestive byproducts and even certain medicines. These free radicals are scavenged by antioxidants. Antioxidants can be obtained through food or supplements. They are also available in anti-ageing serums and creams.

Vitamin C, E, ferulic acid, some minerals such as selenium and chromium, flavonoids found in herbal teas and berries are powerful antioxidants. Blackberries, cranberries, blueberries, beans, artichokes, pecans, walnuts and hazelnuts are foods thought to be the richest in antioxidants.

Also look for antioxidants in your anti-ageing serums and creams. Vitamin C serum is the most popular serum as of today. It gives your skin an extra boost by improving the immune system of the skin, preventing pigmentation, improving skin elasticity, decreasing wrinkles and preventing environmental damage. Choose a vitamin C serum that has L-ascorbic acid and is formulated at a pH range of around 3.5. It should also be packaged in an opaque, air-tight container as vitamin C tends to destabilize on exposure to light and air.

Type	Example
Skin-replenishing	Isdin Ureadin anti-wrinkle melting cream, Avarta anti-ageing cream
Skin-restoring	Sebamed age defense Q10 cream, Yugard cream
Antioxidant	Revibra C10, Flavo C cream

Rapid fire

Question	Answer
What is the right age to start anti-ageing products?	Forty
When do you start anti-ageing skincare?	In your twenties. Be regular with sunscreen and moisturizer.

What about thirties?	Sunscreen, moisturizer and vitamin C or retinoids.
Five anti-ageing products that are important	Sunscreen, moisturizer, retinoid, vitamin C and any anti-ageing ingredient such as peptides, coenzyme Q10, green tea extract, coffee berry, grape seed extract, etc.
Will my skin look like a million bucks if I strictly follow the five-product regime?	Not unless you also eat well, avoid smoking and lead a healthy lifestyle.
Is it true that skincare should begin during childhood?	Yes. Every child above the age of one should be made to wear protective clothing. They should also be moisturized, be it through a daily massage with baby oil or otherwise. Sunscreen can safely be applied on a one-year-old child when outdoors.

When to start treatments

A question I am often asked is, 'When is the right age to start getting Botox or fillers done?' There is no 'right age' for this. Botox is given to children with cerebral palsy and to older people with migraines and eye paralysis. As far as the US FDA is concerned, there is no age restriction for these treatments. The determining factors for anti-ageing treatments are the symptoms, skin conditions and lifestyles of patients. Every doctor has his or her own protocol. To treat a square jaw I inject Botox into the masseter muscle, even for people in their thirties. For wrinkles, I start Botox at thirty-five. I usually give hyaluronic acid fillers for anti-ageing to men and women above forty. But HA fillers for lip plumping or sunken eyes can be given to girls in their late twenties as well. I believe less is more.

Mesotherapy and platelet-rich plasma can be started in one's thirties.

Non-surgical skin tightening with HIFU or radiofrequency can be started as soon as you see your skin beginning to sag. This could be in your late thirties or early forties.

Chemical peels can even be done in your twenties.

Let's see some examples:

1. *Karuna is thirty-five years old. She is beginning to notice laugh lines. Her skin is supple. It can be oily at times. Her pores are looking more prominent. What does she need?*

A.M. routine: An oil-free moisturizer and a sunscreen.
P.M. routine: Antioxidant, like vitamin C serum, at night, followed by a skin-restoring cream, such as a retinol cream, on alternate nights.

2. *Rohan is forty-eight years old. His skin is dry. He has developed a dark band of pigmentation on his forehead. What does he need?*

A.M. routine: A moisturizer and a sunscreen.
P.M. routine: A skin-replenishing cream at night for the full face and an antioxidant cream for his forehead.

3. *Shrividya is fifty-three years old. She is developing lines and wrinkles on her face. Her skin looks blotchy and feels dry. What does she need?*

A.M. routine: A moisturizer and a sunscreen.
P.M. routine: A skin-replenishing cream (e.g. a cream with hyaluronic acid) and a skin-restoring cream (a cream with peptides or coenzyme Q10) at night.

4. *Triveni is gorgeous at sixty-seven years of age. She has no pigmentation. But her skin seems thin and a little dry. She has prominent jowls, neck bands and crow's feet around her eyes and some forehead wrinkles. What does she need?*

A.M. routine: A skin-replenishing cream and an antioxidant, followed by a sunscreen.
P.M. routine: A skin-replenishing cream and a skin-restoring cream at night.

Mickey's mother realized that there was more to a skin routine than cleansing, toning, moisturizing and using a sunscreen. 'Will I look forty-five in four weeks, doc?' she laughed and got up to leave. Adding a few anti-ageing creams that I had prescribed to her otherwise perfect skin routine and healthy lifestyle would surely make her skin look younger, I assured her.

WEEK 4

WEEK 4

12

Food for Skin

'Your diet is a bank account. Good food choices are
good investments'
—Bethenny Frankel

'I think I am a fairly healthy eater,' Mickey said. 'I eat
everything that's available at home and rarely eat out.'
She worked ten hours a day and I was impressed she
carried a lunchbox to work. But her lunch was comprised
of two rotis and a little vegetable. Her dinner again was
rice, dal and a few veggies. No wonder she complained of
hair fall and brittle nails. There was hardly any protein in
her supposedly healthy diet. So we discussed diet.

You can eat your way to healthy skin. Skin and hair
are indeed a manifestation of your overall well-being.

How you feed your body affects your skin too. So if
you want radiant, healthy skin, you better eat right. The
moment your eyes look tired, you develop dark circles or
your cheeks look sunken, your family and friends will say
you look ill. 'Whenever I have submissions in college, it

153

shows on my skin first,' says twenty-one-year-old Ruchika. She works late nights and does not follow a healthy diet. A good diet combined with some dietary supplements can make your skin glow and look younger as well.

'I drink four litres of water a day, but my skin doesn't glow,' says Mona. The skin needs water, proteins, amino acids, vitamins, iron, minerals and fat to function well and look healthy. Human skin is 70 per cent water, 25 per cent protein and 5 per cent fat. This does not mean that if you drink four litres of water, it goes straight to the skin and perks it up. Skin gets its water supply both from inside the body and from the environment outside. Of the 70 per cent water, the outermost layer of the skin, known as the stratum corneum, should contain 10 per cent. This 10 per cent is not obtained from the deeper layers of the skin, as the cells in this layer are dead. They absorb water from the environment. So moisturizing the skin will give the stratum corneum its 10 per cent of water. The remaining 60 per cent is obtained through the intake of about 1.5–2 litres of water a day. Tender coconut water, lemon juice, buttermilk, fruits and vegetables that contain water, such as oranges, grapefruits, strawberries, apples, sprouts, watermelons, lettuce, spinach, cucumbers and tomatoes, also add to the water content of the skin.

Revamping your eating habits can make your skin feel and look like a million bucks. Let us understand the skin nutrients better.

Proteins

'Protein is King'—Dr Spencer Nadolsky

Collagen fibres are the pillars of our skin. They give it its basic form. Collagen is made of fibrous protein and comprises 30 per cent of the total body protein. Our hair, nails and dead skin layer are made up of a protein called keratin. Our muscles and bones are also made of protein. With age, the collagen fibres shrink and degenerate. This results in wrinkles and loose skin. Along with that, muscles and bones are almost eaten up due to loss of protein. This makes the face look like an inverted pyramid, or a bulldog. 'Doctor, I feel like my entire face is drooping,' say my patients who are in their mid-forties and above. So if you want to delay the process of ageing on your face and want your hair to be your crowning glory and your nails to be strong, make sure your protein intake is adequate. Proteins also keep your muscles and bones strong, preventing early ageing.

Sources

Chicken, eggs, lean meat, tofu, soy, Greek yogurt, milk, cheese, French beans, kidney beans, mushrooms, almonds and pure oats.

Daily requirement

An average male with a sedentary lifestyle needs 60 g and an average female with a sedentary lifestyle requires 55 g of protein per day.

Essential fatty acids

Fats are not always the bad guys. I love my teaspoon of organic ghee every day. I just feel it makes my skin *googly woogly woosh*!

'But, doc, won't it make me put on weight? They are fats after all,' ask most of my patients. Not at all. Essential fatty acids are the good fats. The last thing they would make you do is put on weight. They comprise of two groups, omega-3 fatty acids, which originate from linolenic acid, and omega-6 fatty acids, which originate from linoleic acid.

Omega-3 fatty acids are the soldiers who prevent inflammation and fight against it. They help the skin heal faster for those who suffer from acne, eczema or rosacea. Omega-6 fatty acids are the guardian soldiers. They form a protective barrier on the skin's surface. As it is the cell membrane that holds water in, the stronger that barrier is the better your cells can hold moisture. So omega-6 fatty acids make the skin look plump and radiant.

Sources

Omega-3 fatty acids, as well as omega-6 fatty acids, are found in nuts, seeds, oils such as flaxseed oil, canola oil, hemp seed oil, and cold-water fish like salmon and trout.

Daily requirement

There is no official recommendation but a healthy adult usually requires 250–500 mg of essential fatty acids per day. Higher amounts, up to 1500 mg, are recommended for dry skin, eczemas, heart disorders and other health conditions.

Vitamins

'If you don't eat vegetables, you won't get your vitamins!' All of us have heard this in school when we refused to eat our greens. It is, in fact, true. Let's look at the vitamins that are essential for our skin's well-being.

Vitamin C

It is a powerful antioxidant, most prevalent in the skin. It is easily leached away by environmental stress. Exposure from the ozone of city pollution can decrease the level of vitamin C in skin by 55 per cent. Sun exposure and smoking can reduce it by 30 per cent. When taken orally in the form of L-ascorbic acid, vitamin C nudges the skin cells to produce more collagen. It helps heal wounds and prevents discolouration. It functions as an antioxidant by scavenging and quenching free radicals and regenerating vitamin E from its radical form. So if you want to combat pigmentation, tanning and fine lines with one vitamin, this is your superstar.

Oral vitamin C is necessary to prevent scurvy, a disease with many manifestations including gingivitis (swollen and bleeding gums), skin fragility and corkscrew hair, often noticed as dry and splitting hair.

Sources

Oranges, limes, lemons, kiwis, strawberries, raspberries, gooseberries, blueberries, cranberries, cherries, pineapples, mangoes, grapefruits, papayas, guavas, lychees, cantaloupes, tomatoes, kale, broccoli, cauliflowers and red and green peppers.

Daily requirement

For men, 90 mg a day, and for women, 75 mg a day. Smokers need 35 mg more vitamin C per day than non-smokers. However, in cases of pigmentation or skin conditions, an adult would need 1000 mg of vitamin C per day.

Who should not take vitamin C

In a study published in the *Journal of the American Medical Association*, taking more than 7000 mg of vitamin C per week can increase the risk of kidney stones if one has a medical history related to it. Kidney stones are often composed of calcium oxalate. And when excess vitamin C is excreted by the body, it is usually in the oxalate form. This may lead to the formation of stones in the kidney. The caution applies only to vitamin C supplements and not to vitamin C found in food.*

Vitamin E

Vitamin E is a lipid-soluble vitamin that stabilizes the cell membranes of skin against damage by the harmful free fatty acids and phospholipids. It regenerates its

---

* L.D. Thomas et al., 'Ascorbic Acid Supplements and Kidney Stone Incidence among Men: A Prospective Study', *JAMA Internal Medicine* 173 (2013): 386–88.

antioxidant capabilities in the presence of vitamin C. Hence, vitamin C and E work synergistically to fight free radicals. When I go out on holidays, I always take my vitamin C and E supplement; together they fight the harmful effects of UV rays better. In fact, those with skin allergies and eczemas should also opt for this combination because together they have better skin repair capabilities too.

Several studies have shown that vitamin E, when applied on the skin, can reduce damage caused by sun exposure and limit the chances of skin cancer.

If your nails feel lustreless or chip away, just break a vitamin E capsule and apply a few drops of the oil from the capsule on your nails. You can do the same for chapped lips. Vitamin E hydrates and protects your nail cuticle much as it hydrates chapped lips.

Sources

Wheat germ oil, safflower oil, palm oil, sunflower seeds, wheat germ oil, hazelnuts, almonds, pistachios, peanuts, spinach, oats, sweet potatoes, avocados and dairy products.

Daily requirement

One needs 15 mg of vitamin E per day. The most active form of vitamin E is alpha tocopherol. When taken orally, it is known to reduce wrinkles, prevent sun damage and improve skin texture. To be in the safe zone, stay within 400 IU per day or less.

Who should not take vitamin E

Vitamin E can increase the tendency to bleed in an individual. So people on aspirin and other blood thinners should avoid taking it on a daily basis.

Vitamin A

Just like cracks that develop in an old wall or a poorly made foundation, elastin and collagen fibres get damaged due to UV rays, smoking and other unhealthy lifestyle habits. The skin begins to loosen and wrinkles develop. Vitamin A is like a mason who repairs the skin. It helps promote new collagen formation and repairs the skin tissue. Skin tends to get dry and flaky when vitamin A levels are low. So if want your skin to smoothen and your fine lines to reduce, make sure you take enough vitamin A in your food. Vitamin A also protects us from UV rays and infections. It is used to treat skin conditions such as eczema, psoriasis, acne and lichen planus pigmentosus. Lack of vitamin A results in thick, dry skin that is often compared to toad skin.

Sources

Carrots, sweet potatoes, kale, pumpkins, mangoes, spinach, greens and tomatoes.

Daily requirement

2000–3000 IU per day.

Vitamin B3 (Niacinamide)

My mother had pigmentation on her cheeks and she would try every cream that promised to make it disappear. The most popular one in those times was a cream which had niacinamide as its main ingredient.

Niacinamide is another name for vitamin B3 and it has anti-inflammatory and healing properties. It helps the body perform critical functions like DNA repair and is a cellular energy precursor. It decreases water loss through the epidermis and protects the skin barrier, thus keeping the skin supple.

Vitamin B3 also regulates sebum formation in the skin and is known to reduce pigmentation. It can be taken as a supplement orally. It is popularly used in creams to reduce blemishes, pigmentation, fine lines and wrinkles, and to hydrate the skin.

Sources

Legumes, nuts, grain products, mushrooms, chicken, pork and fish.

Daily requirement

One needs 14–16 mg of vitamin B3 per day.

Vitamin B7 (Biotin)

Everybody who has hair loss thinks biotin is the miracle supplement which will arrest the hair fall and make it grow back abundantly. This is not true, because there can be many reasons for hair loss. Nutritional deficiency—in the form of lack of iron, biotin, vitamin D3, proteins, minerals—is only one of the reasons for hair fall. Nonetheless, biotin forms the basis of hair, nails and skin cells, and its deficiency can result in hair loss, brittle nails and itchy, scaly skin.

Sources

Bananas, eggs, oatmeal and rice.

Daily requirement

One needs 5 mg of biotin per day.

Minerals

Most of us don't need to supplement our mineral intake, particularly if we already take a multivitamin. And those who drink spring water, which often contains a natural supply of important minerals, meet their requirement easily. Studies show that washing your face with mineral water can help reduce many common skin irritations. Plus the mineral content helps the skin cells absorb moisture better. The top three minerals needed for skin are selenium, zinc and copper. Chromium and magnesium are needed for people with insulin resistance and PCOS.

Selenium

This is a super antioxidant mineral. It plays an important role in DNA synthesis and repair.

Selenium protects the skin from the harmful effects of UV rays, and also preserves tissue elasticity and slows down the hardening of tissues associated with oxidation.

Sources

Wholegrain cereals, seafood, garlic and eggs.

Daily requirement

55 μg for men and women nineteen years and older.

Zinc

Zinc is an essential trace element in the skin's dietary defense squad. It reduces the formation of free radicals, improves skin immunity, reduces inflammation and helps in the normal healing of wounds. Zinc also regulates cell turnover and reduces the amount of natural oil produced by skin. It is often given as a supplement to improve eczemas, acne, alopecia, scaly skin and seborrheic dermatitis.

Sources

Nuts, beans, fortified cereals, oysters, meat.

Daily requirement

One needs 8 mg of zinc per day.

Copper

This is a trace mineral found naturally in soil. Copper has antibacterial and anti-inflammatory properties. It aids in the repair of wounds and skin that has been cut, abraded or infected. It also rejuvenates the skin by contributing to the formation of new skin cells.

Sources

Seafood, meat, grains, nuts and seeds.

Daily requirement

900 µg per day for men and women above nineteen years of age.

Iron

Iron deficiency can result in hair loss, dark circles and pale skin.

Sources

Eggs, meat, fish, whole grains, dried apricots, prunes and raisins, nuts, seeds, fortified cereals, spinach and beetroot.

Daily requirement

18–20 mg per day.

Beyond vitamins and minerals: The new skin nutrients

Some of the newer, more exciting skin research looks beyond vitamins and minerals. It talks of other nutrients that, when taken internally or applied topically, can have remarkable effects on the skin.

Alpha-lipoic acid

This is a powerful antioxidant for ageing skin which helps scour free radicals from your blood. With the ability to penetrate both oil and water, affecting skin cells inside and on the surface, it is a vital nutrient. Alpha-lipoic acid helps neutralize skin cell damage caused by free radicals. It also helps other vitamins work effectively to rebuild skin cells damaged by environmental assaults, such as smoke and pollution.

Polyphenols

Curcumin

The first time I learnt to ride a bicycle, my excitement knew no bounds. Confident of being able to ride it without support, I went down a slope one day, not realizing that I would end up in the gutter. I got abrasions all over my arms and legs. My mom was extremely worried, but my grandma simply made a paste of turmeric and tulsi leaves and applied it on all my skin wounds. I remember howling as the turmeric paste was being applied because it stung the hell out of me. But it worked like magic. All my wounds healed within two to three days and there was not a scar anywhere on my body. Turmeric has been an integral part of our ancient home remedies. It has existed in Ayurvedic and Chinese medicine for more than 4000 years.

Curcumin is an antioxidant derived from turmeric. It is an anti-inflammatory and anti-carcinogenic polyphenol. It helps to repair skin and heals wounds. It helps prevent lines and wrinkles and makes the skin look youthful.

Sources

Turmeric.

Daily requirement

2–8 g per kg of one's body weight daily.

Green tea

Green tea contains epigallocatechin gallate (EGCG), the most potent tea polyphenol. Again, it is a powerful antioxidant that helps delay the signs of ageing in skin. Green tea does contain caffeine and can affect your sleep. Hence it is better to take it during the day. I love my iced green tea. I add a quarter teaspoon of honey, half a lemon and a few drops of juice extracted from ginger to the tea. Lemon not only gives it tanginess, it also has vitamin C. Honey compensates for sugar and ginger adds the zing and is antibacterial too. It is a perfect replacement for drinks which contain caffeine, sugar and milk.

Sources

Camellia sinensis plant.

Daily requirement

300 mg EGCG per day (4–5 large cups of green tea per day).

Who should not take green tea

If you are pregnant or breastfeeding, you should limit your caffeine intake to less than 200 mg per day. If you are suffering from high blood pressure, heart conditions, bleeding disorders, anaemia, glaucoma or are taking oestrogen or birth control pills, or amphetamines, you should avoid drinking green tea.

Resveratrol

Also known as the fountain of youth, resveratrol is a polyphenol that is produced naturally by several plants either in response to injury or when the plant is under attack by pathogens such as bacteria or fungi. It has potent anti-inflammatory, antioxidant, anti-ageing, anti-acne and skin-lightening properties. It also helps prevent skin cancer. 'If you do not want wrinkles, drink a glass of red wine every day,' said my friend Yashita on a girls' night out. While red wine does have the benefits of resveratrol, it also has the perils of sugar on the skin. So you will have to take Yashita's advice with a pinch of salt.

Sources

Abundant in *Vitis vinifera* (grapevine) and its derivatives (e.g. red wine, purple grape juice), various berries, peanuts, jackfruit and pomegranate.

Daily requirement

100–200 mg of resveratrol daily.

Polypodium leucotomos

A robust antioxidant, it also provides protection against sun rays. Take it on a trip to the beach and I promise you, you will not tan, provided you also apply your sunscreen. It is a perfect oral sunscreen. It is also used to treat skin disorders such as psoriasis, atopic dermatitis, polymorphic light eruption and melasma.

Source

It is an extract obtained from a species of fern called *Polypodiaceae* available in Central and South America. It is not found in food.

Daily requirement

The regular dose is two capsules, one in the morning—thirty minutes before sun exposure—and one before midday. During a vacation, it is better to take two capsules of 300 mg in the morning and two capsules three hours after the morning dose.

Glutathione

It is a fabulous antioxidant that is also used to treat liver toxicity. It prevents melanin formation and reduces its presence in the skin, resulting in lighter and brighter skin. It has been studied for the treatment of autoimmune disorders, such as psoriasis, lichen planus, alopecia areata and polymorphic light eruption, with positive results.

Sources

Tomatoes, avocados, oranges, walnuts and asparagus.

Daily requirement

20–40 mg per day.

Red flag

Glutathione has been doing the rounds for the past couple of years as a skin-whitening agent. People think of it as a wonder drug that can turn you into Cinderella overnight. Of late, large doses of glutathione have been given orally or intravenously without any safety studies or research. Although the recommended dose is 20–40 mg for every kg body weight per day, there are pharmaceutical companies claiming to manufacture up to 50,000 mg of glutathione per injection. This sounds impossible. Safety is also a big concern, as there are no relevant studies involving such large doses of the drug. And don't forget that anything in excess is unsafe and can be toxic to the liver or kidneys.

Carotenoids

Carotenoids are a large family of red, orange and yellow substances found in plants that perform vital antioxidant roles when ingested.

They are the original antioxidants and the most potent free radical scavengers. They protect the skin from damage by skin saboteurs such as sun, stress, pollution, environmental toxins, nicotine, alcohol, etc. Humans and animals cannot synthesize carotenoids, so they must obtain them via ingestion of foods or supplements. The four major dietary carotenoids are carotene, lycopene, lutein and zeaxanthin.

β-Carotene

β-Carotene is a precursor to vitamin A.

Sources

Carrots, bell peppers, mangoes and papayas.

Lutein and Zeaxanthin

These two fighters prevent sun damage. Studies have shown that on ingesting oral supplements of these two carotenoids every day for twelve weeks, there was a significant improvement in skin tone, luminance and colour. Other studies have shown that lutein and zeaxanthin protect keratinocytes from UV radiation–induced skin ageing.

Sources

Green leafy vegetables, such as spinach and kale, and egg yolks.

Daily requirement

6–10 mg a day of lutein and 2 mg a day of zeaxanthin.

Astaxanthin

This carotenoid is said to reduce inflammation and oxidation in the skin. Its cell membrane is composed of two external lipid layers, making it a stronger antioxidant than vitamin E. It is both water and oil soluble, only produced by algae when exposed to intense UV radiation.

There is not enough research on this carotenoid yet, but it is unsafe to take during pregnancy. It should also be avoided by people with hormonal issues, low calcium and osteoporosis.

Sources

One of the largest sources of astaxanthin is certain types of marine algae. It is also found in seafood such as salmon, rainbow trout, shrimp and lobster.

Daily requirement

2–4 mg per day.

Lycopene

This is a potent carotenoid found in most red-coloured fruits and vegetables like tomatoes, watermelons, pink grapefruit, papaya, red bell pepper and pink guava.

Daily requirement

About 5–6 mg per day is sufficient for an adult.

Antioxidants

Everybody talks about them. On asking people what they understand by the word antioxidant, you will get answers like 'They help detox' or 'They purify the blood.'

The body produces free radicals due to internal release of toxins and external agents such as pollution, smoking, alcohol, sun exposure and smog. Free radicals speed up the process of ageing internally in the body organs and externally on the skin's surface. They gobble up collagen and elastin, the fibres that support skin structure. This causes wrinkles and other signs of ageing. Antioxidants protect against DNA damage and prevent free radicals from harming cells in the body and the skin. To sum up, skin plays a major role in the immune system of our body. It is like the head bouncer which protects any attack on the body from pollutants, germs, bacteria and allergens.

Antioxidants are the junior bouncers who aid the head bouncer in its work.

Vitamin C and E and selenium are amongst the top three antioxidants found in food and food supplements. They help the skin look youthful.

Role	Common sources
Antioxidants	Blackberries, blueberries, strawberries, plums
Anti-ageing	Grapes, purple grape juice, berries, jackfruit, pomegranate
Skin-replenishing	Sunflower seeds, hazelnuts, almonds, pistachios, peanuts, spinach, oats, sweet potato, avocado
Skin-hydrating	Chia sees, flax seeds, sunflower seeds, pumpkin seeds, walnuts, fish
Skin-brightening	Oranges, limes, lemon, kiwis, strawberries, raspberries, gooseberries, blueberries, cranberries, cherries, pineapple, mangoes, grapefruit, papayas, guavas, lychees, tomatoes, kale
Skin fighters	Nuts, green leafy vegetables, beans, fortified cereals, oysters, meat
Acne- and blackhead-minimizing	Bitter gourd, green gourd, turmeric
Sunscreen	Carrots, all berries and pomegranate
Building blocks	Chicken, eggs, kidney beans, chickpeas, sprouts, mushrooms, lentils

Now that we know who the good guys are, it is important for us to know the bad ones too.

My grandfather passed away when he was eighty-six years old. He was fit as a fiddle till his last day. At eighty-six, he barely looked seventy. He had salt-and-pepper hair, few wrinkles and a fairly chiselled face. Except for some joint pains, my grandfather had no ailments. He ate vegetables, fruits, legumes, eggs, yogurt, nuts and ghee every day. And I never saw him eat sweets, bread, butter or red meat. He did not smoke or drink alcohol. He went for a walk every morning and evening and was in bed by 10 p.m. every night. He had no bad guys to damage his skin. His good guys were *whole foods*.

On the other hand, my friend Anna went to Atlanta for further studies after twelfth grade. She studied for sixteen hours a day, did no exercise, lived on pizza, chocolate and burgers, and barely slept. Anna is thirty-five years old now but looks fifty-five. High carb foods coupled with a sedentary lifestyle are the reasons for this. Our parents always discouraged us from having junk food. And now I know why.

Sugar and skin

This is an obviously unhealthy combination. Chocolates, ice creams, cakes, sweets, pastries, biscuits, doughnuts, sweetened drinks and alcohol can be delectable to the palate. But they are good for neither the waistline nor the skin. Sugar triggers a process called glycation. Here, sugar molecules bind to collagen and elastin fibres and form advanced glycation end-products (AGEs). This destroys the collagen and elastin fibres, resulting in premature wrinkles, fine lines and uneven skin tones. So think carefully the next time you reach for your sugar fix.

AGEs also increase with grilling, frying, and roasting food. Methods of preparation that are water-based, such as boiling and steaming, produce smaller amounts of AGEs.

Some spices, like cinnamon, cloves, oregano, ginger and garlic, inhibit the endogenous production of AGEs and are worth adding to your food to prevent early skin ageing.

High glycaemic index food

Food with glycaemic indexes above seventy increase the production of insulin in the body. High insulin levels result in inflammation, resistance to insulin's ability to store sugar and weight gain. This elevates hormones that increase the activity of sebaceous glands in the skin and the formation of acne. White bread, white rice cakes, instant oats, white potatoes, most crackers, bagels, cakes, doughnuts, croissants, biscuits, sweets and most packaged breakfast cereals are foods with high glycaemic indexes. They should be avoided.

Avoiding sugar is understandable. But why do most dermatologists and nutritionists ask you to forgo dairy as well?

Presently, milk is sourced from pregnant dairy cows who have been pumped with antibiotics and hormones to secrete more milk. The milk produced has high levels of circulating progesterone, insulin-like growth factor and other hormones which, when ingested, convert into dihydrotestosterone (DHT). These hormones send the oil glands into overdrive, triggering acne in susceptible people. They can also give rise to hives and allergies.

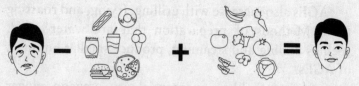

Subtract the bad and add the good food to look youthful

Probiotics

Considering the high usage of pesticides in agriculture and the reduction of the normal protective bacterial flora in our gut, probiotic has become a fast-emerging dietary recommendation.

Probiotics are a group of microorganisms living within our bodies and on our skin. There are over 10,000 different types of microorganisms living inside us. They are essential for the proper functioning of our body and skin. Each of us have our own complex array of probiotics. This is called our microbiome.

It was recently discovered that skin has its own microbiome. It is primarily composed of bacteria, but also includes fungi, viruses and protozoa. A microbiome protects our skin from allergens, oxidative damage and harmful bacteria such as *Staphylococcus aureus* and Group A streptococcus. It also inhibits inflammation and stimulates the production of antimicrobial peptides that kill harmful bacteria, fungi and viruses.

Yogurt, yakult, kimchi, kefir fermented food and apple cider vinegar are probiotics that we take orally to keep our gut healthy. They keep the bad bugs away and ensure that the good bugs stay. Our skin microbiome plays the same role of determining which bacteria is a friend and which one a foe. However, when the bad bacteria are higher in number than the good bacteria, they wreak havoc on the skin. They also stimulate the good bacteria, making them multiply. And as you know, anything in excess is bad. So these good bacteria can now result in rosacea, acne, etc.

Probiotics are now available in cream formulations too. However, due to their inherent instability, light and air cause them to break down faster. Hence, they should not be packaged in jars. A probiotic cream should contain a mix of probiotics, lysate ingredients and prebiotics (to fuel the probiotics). These help improve the immunity of the skin. Lactobacillus, Bifidobacterium, Vitreoscilla and various prebiotic sugars such as xylitol and fructooligosaccharides are ingredients you should look for in probiotic creams.

Probiotic creams restore the pH balance of the skin. They keep the skin hydrated and protect it from environmental threats.

There is so much about food and skin that I could go on writing pages. But this was the essential gist of it all. Mickey said it was an eye-opener for her as she had always been under the impression that she ate healthy. She said she would now add a fair amount of protein to her diet. She would drink two litres of water every day and eat all the brightly coloured fruits and vegetables. 'Not the artificially coloured ones, doc, I shall only buy organic stuff,' she said aloud while getting into her car. 'Yes, and don't forget the best diet is a protein-rich, sugar-free, low-salt diet with a small amount of carbs and a little bit of essential fats too,' I hollered back.

13

Exercise and Your Skin

'To enjoy the glow of good health, you must exercise'

—Gene Tunney

'I don't have time for exercise but I do walk for about ten minutes from my house to the bus stop every morning and evening,' Mickey said. Exercise is essential and twenty minutes of routine walk was certainly not enough for Mickey. I asked her to try going for a brisk walk or a jog for at least half an hour every day. An even better option would be to join a dance class. It would be like killing two birds with one stone—get the daily exercise and become party-ready too.

While some people exercise to lose weight, others exercise to keep fit and increase their stamina. Exercise also helps the heart and other organs to function well.

A stealthier pay-off to why you should stick to your New Year's resolution of hitting the gym every day is healthy skin. Haven't you noticed how your skin looks when you are blushing and how it glows after a run? This is because exercise improves circulation. This allows more nutrients and oxygen to reach your skin, while removing toxins and waste products more efficiently.

Skin cells contain organelles called mitochondria. Mitochondria are the work engines that generate energy. They help the skin repair itself from sun damage and other external assaults. They also help build collagen. Research has shown that exercise boosts these mitochondria, along with toning the skin and making it tauter. It also inhibits the villainous free radicals and improves the activities of antioxidants in the skin. It also prevents the process of glycation in the cells. Together, this helps prevent premature ageing of the skin.[*]

Exercise also ensures better sleep, thereby benefitting the skin indirectly. Unhealthy sleep patterns and insufficient sleep cause early ageing of the skin, resulting in dark circles, fine lines and dullness.

In addition, exercise reduces the level of cortisol and releases endorphins. This in turn can lower stress and fight skin aliens such as hives, acne, dullness, etc.

---

[*] C. Couppe, R.B. Svensson, J.F. Grosset, V. Kovanen, R.H. Nielsen, M.R. Olsen et al., 'Life-long Endurance Running Is Associated with Reduced Glycation and Mechanical Stress in Connective Tissue', *Age (Dordrecht, Netherlands)* 36 (2014): 9665.

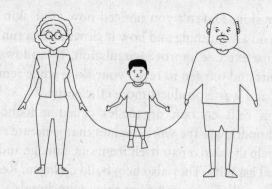

Exercise

Pre-workout skincare

Wash you face well. Remove all make-up. It is a bad idea to wear make-up while exercising. Sweat infused with make-up clogs the pores and gives rise to acne or whiteheads.
Apply a good moisturizer. You sweat as you exercise. This dehydrates the body as well as the skin. So you need to hydrate your skin in advance. If you take spinning or hot yoga classes, use a thicker moisturizer.
If it's an outdoor workout, do not forget to use sunscreen on your face, neck and arms.
Carry wet wipes with you. Clean the workout equipment you plan to use to prevent bacteria from infecting your skin.
If you are swimming, use a waterproof sunscreen and a moisturizer.
During your workout, wipe off sweat with a clean towel.
Drink a lot of water.
Use a thermal water mist while doing weights or cardio. This will clean your skin, clear the sweat and purify it with rich minerals.

Post workout

First wash your hands. They must be dirty with a mixture of sweat, dirt and microorganisms from all the equipment you have used.
Next, splash water on your face.
Take a shower. Cleanse well to remove all the sweat, bacteria and grime from your scalp and body. This will prevent acne and body odour.
Change into a fresh pair of clothes. Dump the sweaty clothes and socks in your washing machine. Do not wear them again without washing. Dirty clothes harbour fungi and bacteria.
Apply a generous amount of moisturizer on your face and body.
Have a protein-rich diet to prevent hair loss.

One of my close friends is a renowned Pilates instructor. She has never had the need to do any skin treatments on her face. All she does is use a sunscreen in the day and a vitamin C serum and retinol cream at bedtime. Sometimes she teases me saying I purposely don't inject Botox and fillers into her face because I want to look younger than her. At any given time of the year, her skin looks amazing. The rewards of exercise are not just a healthy body but also radiant skin.

So instead of ditching your workout because you don't have the time, *make* time for it!

14

Home Remedies

'Beware of false knowledge. It is more dangerous than ignorance'

—George Bernard Shaw

'My granny's skin is still so smooth and beautiful, doc. You know, she is eighty years old but she doesn't look a day older than seventy,' said Mickey. Genes, lifestyle and good skincare is the secret.

My granny used to apply coconut oil on her face and entire body every day after her bath. She was using a natural organic moisturizer. Coconut oil is rich in lauric acid and has antibacterial properties. Hence it keeps the skin moisturized and germ-free. I'm sure she didn't know the significance of trapping the skin moisture after bath but she did it right. She had her own set of home-made packs. I think she applied every leftover raw vegetable and fruit on her face. In other words, she was doing her own peels at home. Fruit and vegetable extracts have a lot of acids like glycolic, citric, lactic acids which must have worked on her skin to destroy the bad pigment and keep her collagen fibres strong. And what better exfoliant than the powdered pulses she used to scrub her face with. Even today, herbs, flowers and fruits play a big role in skincare.

'Ghee in my coffee has also shown a huge improvement in making my skin look naturally moisturized,' says actor Jacqueline Fernandez. Actor Richa Chadha swears by natural packs. 'I have always tried to be as natural as possible, given that our profession demands we use a lot of make-up at all times. I use besan and multani mitti packs for instant lifts,' she says.

Let us look at some do-it-yourself tricks to keep your skin radiant and healthy.

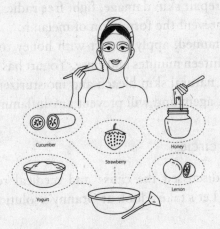

Home remedies

For tan removal

Our skin has its own defence mechanisms. Melanin, the pigment which gives skin its colour, protects the skin from UV rays. This is why dark-skinned people rarely get sun burns or skin cancer. When we are out in the sun for long hours, UV rays trigger the melanocytes present in the skin to produce more melanin. It's the body's way of protecting the skin. This results in a tan. A tan goes off by itself in about eight to twelve weeks. But if you continue to be out in the sun, a tan could persist. Sheets of melanin are laid down, leading to pigmentation.

Tips from the kitchen

The Chinese apply cooled black tea on sunburnt skin for ten to fifteen minutes. Tannic acid, theobromine and catechins repair skin damage, fight free radicals, cool the skin and prevent the formation of melanin.

Once tanned, apply yogurt with honey to your skin for ten to fifteen minutes and rinse. Yogurt has lactic acid, which is a natural skin bleach and moisturizer. Honey is a soothing agent and will prevent any inflammation.

For dark circles

We have discussed the cause and medical remedies in chapter 7. Let's take a look at Granny's solution for dark circles.

Tips from the kitchen

Take two almonds and crush them to make a paste. Add three to four drops of milk and apply this paste under the eyes for fifteen to twenty minutes daily. Almonds contain vitamin E, which hydrates the skin. Both milk and almonds help lighten the skin.

Prepare fresh cucumber juice. Drink some of it and keep the rest in the freezer for fifteen minutes. Place soft cotton soaked in chilled cucumber juice under the eyes for a few minutes. Cucumber juice contains ascorbic acid oxidase, which makes it a good astringent. It is also a mild diuretic when taken orally. Hence, it soothes the skin, reduces puffiness and makes the dark circles appear less prominent.

Apple, again, can be effective against dark circles. Cut thin slices of the fruit and leave them under the eyes for a few minutes. Apple contains tannins that help diminish dark circles. In addition, it has potassium and water-soluble vitamins like B and C that restore lost nutrients to the under-eye skin.

For acne

I often see girls and boys applying lemon juice, tomato and even garlic paste on their pimples. These are highly acidic and can cause irritation. They can also leave burns, blemishes and ugly scars on the skin.

Toothpaste can also cause an irritant reaction.

Tips from the kitchen

Make a paste of neem leaves. Add half a teaspoon of honey to it. Apply this on the pimples for ten minutes. Rinse with cold water. Honey has been used topically for centuries to heal wounds and burns. In vitro, honey has been found to carry out antibacterial and antifungal activity against organisms that commonly infect surgical wounds. Neem leaves have antimicrobial effects and will kill the germs that cause acne. They also help cleanse the skin.

Tea tree oil, an essential oil extracted from the leaves of *Melaleuca alternifolia*, a small tree indigenous to Australia, is also beneficial. It reduces blackheads and whiteheads as well as dryness, itching and burning. It can be applied once a day and left on for about four hours and should then be washed. Tea tree oil is also used as an astringent or a toner.

Witch hazel (*Hamamelis virginiana*) bark extract is considered very safe for topical use as an acne treatment.[*] A decoction can be made with 5 gm of the herb in one cup of water, and then applied on the affected area. It should be left for about twenty minutes and then rinsed. Green tea bags can also be applied on acne. Tannins present in green tea and witch hazel have natural astringent, anti-inflammatory and antiseptic properties.

Dark elbows and knees

Constant friction, like when we rest our elbows on the table while sitting, while kneeling down, even in our denims, can result in the darkening of elbows and knees.

---

[*] A. Peirce, ed., *The American Pharmaceutical Association Practical Guide to Natural Medicines* (New York: Stonesong Press Inc., 1999).

Tips from the kitchen

Take two teaspoons of chickpea and make a paste. Add a pinch of turmeric and a tablespoon of yogurt. Apply this mixture to the elbows, knees, knuckles and ankles. Leave this on for thirty minutes and then wash thoroughly. Immediately dab a moisturizer on slightly damp skin. Do this every alternate day for a couple of weeks to reduce the dark colour. Make sure you do not wear clothes that are tight on your elbows and knees. Chickpea is a good cleanser, yogurt is a moisturizer and skin lightener, and turmeric is an antiseptic.

Make a paste of masoor dal (orange lentil flour). Add half a teaspoon of lemon juice and one teaspoon of tomato juice to one tablespoon of the masoor dal paste. Add a pinch of turmeric, and apply this on the elbows and knees. Leave it for fifteen minutes and then wash it off with cool water.

For cracked feet

My mom always had cracks on her heels. At times, they would bleed. Cracks occur on the feet if you walk barefoot, stand for long hours or wear ill-fitting shoes. They also happen if you use harsh soaps that strip your skin of natural oils.

Tips from the kitchen

Add a tablespoon of almond oil to half a bucket of lukewarm water. Soak your feet in the water for not more than five to seven minutes. Scrub the dead skin with a pumice stone. Apply fresh aloe vera gel to your feet after rinsing them. Aloe vera gel is obtained from the central core of the leaf and has been used topically for centuries to treat wounds and burns. It is anti-inflammatory, hydrating, and also helps cracks heal fast. You can leave the aloe vera on for an hour. Wipe it off instead of rinsing it away. 'Applying aloe vera on my skin also works like magic,' says actor Elli Avram.

For instant glow

When you have a party to attend and no time to visit a skin clinic or get a facial, don't worry. Your skin can still look like a million bucks with a simple home-made mask.

Tips from the kitchen

Pomegranate mask: Prepare fresh pomegranate juice. Drink the juice, but don't throw the pulp away. Instead, add honey and yogurt and make it into a paste. Use this as a face pack after cleansing your skin. Leave it on for twenty minutes and rinse. Your skin will look bright and beautiful with this instant-glow pack. Pomegranate is loaded with antioxidants like flavonoids and phenolics. It also has high levels of vitamins A, E and C. Thus, it delays premature ageing and lightens the skin tone.

Papaya mask: Take a small piece of ripe papaya and a quarter of a cucumber. Make a puree of both. Add a tablespoon of yogurt. Refrigerate this mixture for an hour so that it thickens. Finally, add a teaspoon of honey. Apply it to your face and neck. Leave it on for fifteen minutes and wash. Your skin will look bright and fresh. Papain, the main enzyme in papaya, dissolves the dead skin cells and works as an antibacterial to fight infection. It brightens the skin and makes it more even.

For chapped lips

Dry, chapped lips can be irritating and painful.

Tips from the kitchen

Apply ghee or butter as often as possible. Do *not* lick your lips.

Almond paste or malai can also be applied thrice a day to reduce dryness.

Mix sugar with honey and use it as a gentle scrub to exfoliate dead skin on the lips. Apply coconut oil after exfoliating to lock in moisture and help the lip mucosa heal.

What should one keep in mind before home remedies?
Know your skin type.
If you have dry or flaky skin, or are on acne medication, do not use fruit extracts, potato, tomato juice or lime juice on your skin. These will dehydrate the skin and make it more sensitive. They could even lead to irritation and burns.
If you have oily skin, avoid using malai, milk and oils on your face. These will clog the pores and give rise to more whiteheads.

Ensure that your ingredients are not old. And that the containers as well as the applicators are clean. Otherwise you may develop boils or an infection.
If you have sensitive skin and break into rashes easily, do not try home remedies without consulting a dermatologist. I have seen people break into hives or itchy skin even with aloe vera, honey or yogurt.
Do not try home remedies without having your doctor examine your skin first and give you the green signal.

Now that I have given you some tips, you should also know the pitfalls. People usually love to experiment with home remedies for any ailment, let alone on the skin. With the Internet easily accessible and hundreds of websites providing information on such remedies, the risk of skin allergies, scarring, irritant contact dermatitis and post-inflammatory hyperpigmentation have gone up. People love anything natural even if it is as caustic as lime (calcium hydroxide).

I present to you five cases where people have used home remedies for their skin and developed scars and rashes. These patients used:

- Toothpaste on acne.
- Garlic paste for acne and post-acne pigmentation.
- Calcium hydroxide for earlobe repair.
- Tomato and lemon overnight for dark circles.
- Cinnamon and honey paste for glowing skin.

It is important to know that not every home remedy is safe and not everything you read on the Internet should be believed.

'What should you do if you have an allergic reaction?' Mickey asked.

Apply ice. Take an anti-allergic tablet like Avil. See a dermatologist immediately.

Every skin is unique and will behave differently with the same products or even home remedies. It is best to try the DIY recipes on a small patch first and leave it for at least an hour. If you do not develop any reaction, you can go ahead and use the ingredients on your entire face. Home remedies do help in achieving radiant skin when used the right way for the right skin type. However, you need to understand that not everything is holy grail—a lot can be snake oil too.

WEEK 5

15

Lifestyle and Skin

'The creation of the world did not take place once
and for all time, but takes place every day'
—Samuel Beckett

Although we had had a serious discussion on lifestyle on
the very first day, when I met Mickey at the beginning of
week five, I checked on her to make sure that she had not
touched a cigarette in the past four weeks.

Mickey, I remember, had told me at the beginning
that she led a healthy lifestyle but was an occasional
smoker. When she was stressed, she smoked more. She
also drank a glass of wine twice or thrice a week. It
seemed like she was a happy person with no enemies.
But hold on, she did have some skin enemies and needed
to be aware of them. So I told Mickey a story about my
childhood neighbours.

Riyan and Kian were our neighbours for almost
twelve years and were identical twins. When they were

in school, no one could tell one from the other. To make it more complex, their parents even dressed them alike. As they entered their teens, their interests began to differ. Riyan became a sports lover. He played outdoors all day long—soccer, cricket, hockey—and was a champ. His mom had to scream and yell at him for not bathing even after a game of sweaty soccer.

Kian on the other hand was a computer whiz. He worked on scientific projects over weekends and through his vacations. He was also very particular about his skin and hair. He made sure he used a sunscreen every morning and oiled his hair every Sunday. He even watched his mom apply malai and besan on her face and tried it on himself sometimes. He had read in a magazine that it was not a *girl thing* because men had skin too.

As they entered the work sphere, Riyan quit sports and became a party lover after work. With parties came smoking and alcohol. Kian, on the other hand, loved his sleep and never partied after work. Now both are in their early forties. And you know what, anyone can tell one from the other. Riyan has grey hair, his face looks permanently tanned, he has racoon eyes with wrinkles around them. At forty, he looks fifty-five. Kian, however, looks barely thirty. He is a fairly well-built, tall, fair and handsome guy with dark hair, no wrinkles, no dark circles. Both had the same genes, so what went wrong?

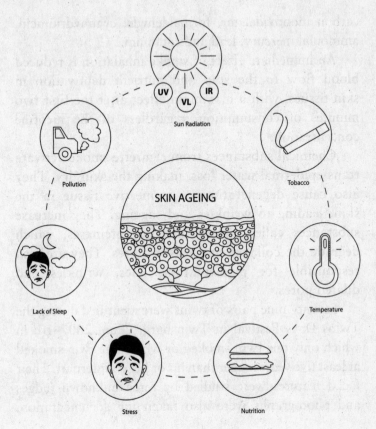

UV   VL   IR

Sun Radiation

Pollution

Tobacco

SKIN AGEING

Lack of Sleep

Temperature

Stress

Nutrition

Enemies of the skin

Smoking and skin

One inhalation from a cigarette contains more than 3800
different harmful, chemical substances, notably nicotine,

carbon monoxide, tar, formaldehyde, cyanhydric acid, ammonia, mercury, lead and cadmium.[*]

An immediate effect of smoke inhalation is reduced blood flow to the skin and nutrient deprivation in skin tissues, with a maximum effect after the first two minutes of consumption, regardless of the nicotine concentration.[†]

Chemical substances from cigarette smoke activate trans-epidermal water loss, making the skin dry. They also cause degeneration of connective tissue in the skin, leading to wrinkles and sagging. They increase substances called matrix metalloproteinases, which degrade the collagen and elastin fibres. They are also responsible for pigmentation, lines, wrinkles and dilated pores.[‡]

Seventy-nine pairs of twins were identified during the Twins Days Festival in Twinsburg, Ohio, 2007–10, in which only one twin smoked or where one twin smoked at least five years longer than his or her counterpart. Their facial features were studied by three unknown judges and photographs were also taken for documentation.

---

[*] H. Bartsch et al., 'Black (Air-cured) and Blond (Flue-cured) Tobacco Cancer Risk IV: Molecular Dosimetry Studies Implicate Aromatic Amines as Bladder Carcinogens', *European Journal of Cancer* 29A (1993): 1199–207.

[†] G. Monfrecola et al., 'The Acute Effect of Smoking on Cutaneous Microcirculation Blood Flow in Habitual Smokers and Nonsmokers', *Dermatology* 197, no. 2 (1998): 115–18.

[‡] L.N. Jorgensen, et al., 'Less Collagen Production in Smokers', *Surgery* 123, no. 4 (April 1998): 450–55; D.P. Kadunce et al., 'Cigarette Smoking: Risk Factor for Premature Facial Wrinkling', *Annals of Internal Medicine* 114 (1991): 840–44.

It was seen that the group which smoked had worse scores when it came to wrinkles around eyes, laugh lines, under-eye puffiness, dark circles and lines around the lips.[*]

In another study, a significant decrease in oxygen content and an increase in temperature were observed in the skin after smoking.[†]

In Mickey's case, she had a few fine wrinkles, and dark circles had begun to appear since she was an occasional smoker. I have seen many patients looking older than their age, all thanks to nicotine. Eric was another groom who came to me just ten days before his wedding and wanted his dark lips to be lightened. It was an impossible task and I had no choice but to let him down by refusing his ten-day challenge. He was a chain-smoker for over three years which had resulted in dark lips and dark gums. I would need at least six to eight months to resolve his issue, provided he quit smoking.

I met my friend Katie for lunch after almost five years. She was my batchmate in college and was this beautiful girl with lovely features. But now she looked haggard and at least ten years older than me. Her face and neck were blotchy, there was a grey tinge to her skin, and her eyes were sunken and dark. Who was the culprit? Cigarette. Katie was a chronic smoker and puffed at least eight cigarettes a day. But now that her

[*] H.C. Okada et al., 'Facial Changes Caused by Smoking: A Comparison between Smoking and Nonsmoking Identical Twins', *Plastic and Reconstructive Surgery* 132, no. 5 (2013): 1085–92.

[†] G.B. Fan et al., 'Changes of Oxygen Content in Facial Skin before and after Cigarette Smoking', *Skin Research and Technology* 18, no. 4 (2012): 511–15.

daughter was going to get married in seven months, she realized she couldn't look like this. I thought it was my duty as a friend and a dermatologist to make the bride's mother look youthful and resplendent at her daughter's wedding. All her skin problems were due to smoking and bad eating habits. For the mornings, I gave her a hyaluronic acid–based cream followed by a sunscreen to apply. At bedtime, I told her to use a vitamin C serum and a cream containing niacinamide, and also prescribed some antioxidant supplements. The most difficult part was convincing her to quit smoking. I had to counsel her for an hour. It wouldn't be easy, I told her, but nothing is impossible if you make up your mind. I asked her to reduce the number of cigarettes she smoked every day gradually, and switch to e-cigarettes, use zero nicotine patches and basically be determined to divert her mind. Katie had seven months, so she could do it. I called her every two weeks to do a yellow peel. Once we finished six peels in three months, I switched to Spectra Revital once a month, which is a laser treatment for pigment reduction. I strictly monitored her smoking habits. One month before the wedding, Katie and her daughter Victoria came in to see me. What a change there was! Both looked like two gorgeous sisters. Katie's sallow skin had now turned into radiant, blemish-free skin. There was hardly any pigmentation and her eyes sparkled and looked bright. 'All my friends want to know what I have been doing because my skin has taken a 180-degree turn to look like this,' Katie said.

Smoking leads to:

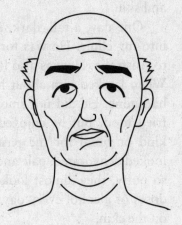

- Dark circles
- Dark lips
- Crow's feet (wrinkles around eyes)
- Fine lines and wrinkles around the lips
- Dull and pale skin
- Stained gums
- Discoloured nails
- Thinning and premature greying of hair
- Hair fall
- Other effects: delayed healing, exacerbation of psoriasis, eczemas, skin cancers, oral cancers and other skin disorders

So the next time you light a cigar, just remember what it's going to do to your skin. It's a war between youthfulness and those few minutes of feeling good and a false perception of stress release.

Alcohol and skin

How can alcohol be bad for skin? Isn't wine an antioxidant?

Not all alcohol is wine, and not all wine is good for the skin.

So let's peep into this relationship between alcohol and skin.

One day, a tall, dark, not so handsome guy walked into my clinic. He was forty and was going to relocate to Australia. He was also looking at marriage proposals. When I asked him about his skincare ritual, he said he had none. He did not smoke, nor did he have sugar or fried food. But he enjoyed his whiskey every night—a kind of ritual for the past four years. No wonder he looked dehydrated, pale and shrunken! And his eyes were so puffy, they almost looked like frog eyes. Even small doses of alcohol every day can have a cumulative effect on the skin.

Alcohol hinders the production of vasopressin, an antidiuretic hormone. Hence, one tends to pee more, which dehydrates the skin, leaving it dry and lustreless. Dry skin in turn leads to rashes, itching, wrinkles, fine lines and loss of resilience.

Alcohol also causes the blood vessels to dilate, causing flushed skin and broken capillaries on the face.

Not only that, alcohol contains destructive molecules called aldehydes, which cause inflammation and cellular damage to the skin cells. This results in enlarged pores, fine lines, sagging skin and discolouration.

Puffy eyes, again, are a result of drinking too much alcohol.

Cocktails have another flipside: sugar. Mojitos and alcohol mixed with sweetened aerated drinks are loaded with sugar, which causes cell damage and skin ageing.

Margaritas taste great but are a double whammy, with both the sugar and the salt in them leading to inflammation as well as bloating and puffiness of eyes or sometimes the entire face.

Different alcohols have different effects on the skin, but as a general rule: the clearer, the better. Vodka, tequilas and gin get flushed out faster. So if you have to drink occasionally, these would be better if you do not want your skin to get damaged, provided you drink in small quantities.

What about wine?

Red wine is rich in antioxidants but causes inflammation too. So it is good in limited quantities. It should be had with a meal to avoid the rapid rise in blood sugar. Red wine can also cause increased flushing due to histamine release in some people. Seventy-six per cent of the people who drink red wine have a flair of their rosacea, versus 56 per cent who drink white wine, 41 per cent who drink beer and 21 per cent scotch drinkers. But the bottom line is, any alcohol will exacerbate rosacea.[*]

Alcohol contains chemical substances called congeners, produced during the fermentation process. Congeners not only contribute to liquors' unique smell and tastes, but they are also responsible for hangovers. So next time you have had a hangover in spite of having

---

[*] H. Alinia et al., 'Rosacea Triggers: Alcohol and Smoking', *Dermatologic Clinics* 36, no. 2 (April 2018): 123–26.

less alcohol, blame it on the congener. And of course, the more the hangover, the more haggard the look.

The best way to combat the ill effects of alcohol is to drink plenty of water. Squeeze an entire lemon into a glass of water and have it as a shot. This will surely neutralize the hangover.

For good skin, train yourself to be a sophisticated party drinker who holds a glass of wine from the beginning of the party to the end.

Stress

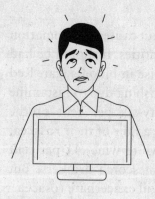 When my uncle developed a rash all over his body and we found no cause for it, I said it could be stress-induced. My uncle laughed and said, 'You dermatologists have one common reason for every ailment. Stress is a part of everyone's life, it is easy for you to blame stress.'

'Srini uncle, it is not a blame game, there is science behind this theory,' I told him.

When we say 'stress', it is always attributed to mental stress and worry pertaining to family or work. A painful situation, fear of something either in college or in office, a remark which feels like a knife piercing through the heart, all these can lead to stress. But what we do not realize is that stress to the body can also be caused due to illness, exertion, overwork, lack of sleep, injury and even extreme temperatures.

When one is stressed, epinephrine and norepinephrine are released from the adrenal glands—the tiny glands sitting on top of our kidneys.

Our body releases cortisol under any stressful circumstance. Cortisol increases the sugar in our blood, which in turn leads to the process of glycation. Glycation damages the collagen and elastin fibres present in the dermis of our skin. When collagen fibres are damaged, the skin becomes lax and fine lines as well as wrinkles appear. When elastin fibres are damaged, the skin loses its ability to bounce back, i.e. it loses its elasticity and suppleness.

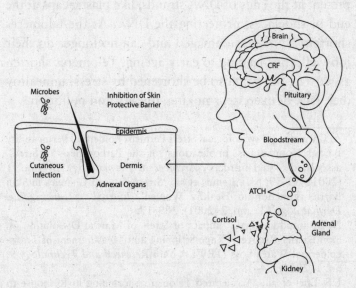

Effect of stress on cortisol

I found some interesting studies where stress due to exams or an interview resulted in raised cortisol levels in blood and a reduction in the skin immunity, as well as a delay in the skin barrier function recovery.[*]

Another study showed that stress due to marital disruption significantly delayed skin barrier recovery.[†]

This indicates that stress can also cause dryness, itching, acne and even exacerbate existing skin disorders such as eczemas, psoriasis, atopic dermatitis, urticaria, etc.

In various other studies, chronic stress such as childhood adversity, nursing elderly dementia parents, special children or chronically ill children, exposure to partner violence, depression can all lead to shortening of telomeres, resulting in premature ageing. Telomeres are present at the ends of DNA strands, like plastic caps at the end of shoelaces, protecting the DNA. As the telomeres shorten, DNA gets damaged and can no longer do their job well, thus leading to early ageing. Telomeres shorten as we age, but can also be shortened by stress, unhealthy diet, lack of exercise, smoking, obesity and pollution.[‡]

---

[*] A. Garg et al., 'Psychological Stress Perturbs Epidermal Permeability Barrier Homeostasis: Implications for the Pathogenesis of Stress-associated Skin Disorders', *Archives in Dermatology* 137, no. 1 (2001): 53–59; M. Altemus et al., 'Stress-induced Changes in Skin Barrier Function in Healthy Women', *Journal of Investigative Dermatology* 117, no. 2 (2001): 309–17.

[†] N. Muizzuddin et al., 'Impact of Stress of Marital Dissolution on Skin Barrier Recovery: Tape Stripping and Measurement of Trans-epidermal Water Loss (TEWL)', *Skin Research and Technology* 9, no. 1 (2003): 34–38.

[‡] E.S. Epel et al., 'Accelerated Telomere Shortening in Response to Life Stress', *Proceedings of the National Academy of Sciences of the United States of America* 101, no. 49 (2004): 17312–15.

Stress also increases the formation of free radicals in the body, including the skin.

If you go back to your chemistry class in eighth grade, free radicals are those unpaired electrons which lie free and fly around looking for another particle to bind with. Once they bind to particles in the skin, they cause oxidation. Oxidation corrupts the skin cells like how iron rusts on exposure to oxygen. Free radicals are formed due to pollution, stress, nicotine, UV rays, alcohol, unhealthy diet, dust and smoke, to name a few.

Has it started sounding like jargon? Well, the long and short of it is that stress can:

- Cause dark circles and baggy eyes
- Cause acne
- Make the skin more sensitive by releasing inflammatory neuropeptides in the skin. This could lead to itching, redness, hives, etc.
- Exacerbate existing skin problems such as psoriasis, eczemas, rosacea, seborrhoeic dermatitis, atopic dermatitis, pruritus and alopecia areata
- Increase oil production, leading to clogged pores, whiteheads and blackheads
- Cause fine lines and wrinkles
- Cause excessive hair loss by speeding up the hair cycle and moving the hair to the telogen (rest) phase
- Speed up greying of the hair

'Who does not have stress?' asks my patient Ritwik. Stress is indeed a part of our lives but the way we deal with it is what matters.

I am neither a motivational speaker nor a wise guru but from experience and practice, I have certainly learnt a few ways to deal with stress:

- No stress is big if you look at the bigger picture. My husband says, stress about something for a day and then leave it, because it is not worth taking the stress if stress isn't the solution to your problem!
- Laugh. Keep away from people who give you stress. Keep away from negativity. Learn to say 'no' when required and do things that make you laugh. The *American Journal of the Medical Sciences* reported a study where participants who watched a comedy video were found to have lower levels of the stress hormones ACTH and cortisol than a control group. So sometimes your WhatsApp forwards may actually do you good by making you laugh.
- Meditate. Ever since I started meditating for twenty minutes every morning, I have been able to cope with stressful situations better. I

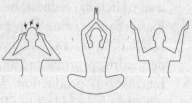

Meditation

find myself calmer and do not get agitated or worried over little things. In a study published in the *Journal of Clinical Psychiatry* in 2013, it was seen that mindfulness meditation lowers anxiety and reduces cortisol levels. Yoga has a meditative component that is particularly effective for reducing stress and lowering cortisol levels.

- Exercise. Weight-bearing exercise such as lifting weights can lower blood sugar levels by making tissues more sensitive to insulin. So they help prevent premature ageing. Exercise also releases a lot of endorphins and norepinephrine, both of which make you feel good.

- Unplug from technology. I have gone off WhatsApp for the past three years and it feels like my biggest achievement. I have also made a rule at home: whenever we go to family dinners, movies or outings, I do not let my family members take their phones. I leave my phone at home too. It is good to unwind and spend some quality time with your family and yourself. Believe me, it is a big stress buster.

- Manage your time. There should be a work–life balance and this comes with discipline and time management. Make sure to keep some leisure time for yourself too. Do not over-schedule your appointments. Do not try to do everything yourself. Learn to trust your staff and colleagues and delegate work. Prioritize your task in such a way that if you leave something out, it doesn't stress you.

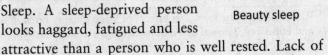

Beauty sleep

- Sleep. A sleep-deprived person looks haggard, fatigued and less attractive than a person who is well rested. Lack of sleep is indirect stress to the body and has its adverse effects on the skin. In a study conducted to check the effects of sleep deprivation, it was seen that people who had a poor quality of sleep showed increased signs of skin ageing such as dark circles, uneven pigmentation, fine lines and reduced elasticity. They also recover much slower if their skin barrier gets disrupted due to other factors.[*]

Once you are stress-free, you will find that your radiance is back, your hair stops falling, your dark circles reduce, your pimples disappear. It just works like magic.

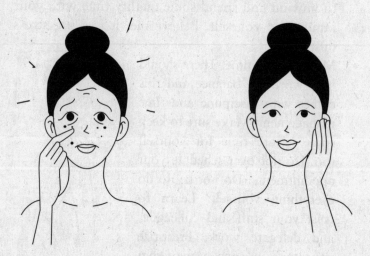

Pimples disappear with reduced stress

[*] P. Oyetakin-White et al., 'In Effects of Sleep Quality on Skin Aging and Function', *Journal of Investigative Dermatology* (2013).

Pollution

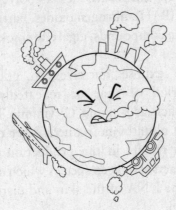

Environmental toxins

I live by the creek of the Arabian sea. Earlier I'd wake up in the morning to the clear blue waters and the stretch of greens. At the far end, I would be able to see the bridge connecting Navi Mumbai to Mumbai and the vehicles would look like tiny toys moving slowly. One look outside my window and there would be happiness on my face. But these days, all I see is a sheet of smog.

For those few hours in the morning, it feels like the sea and the marsh have all migrated to another place and the sky and earth have become one huge mass of grey. This is the pollution from the surrounding industries and the soot from the vehicles.

When I see a man with a band of dark colour on his forehead, I know he is either working as a traffic police officer or spends most of his time either on the streets or in chemical industries.

Do you know that the polluted air we breathe in contains harmful chemicals such as polycyclic aromatic hydrocarbons (PAH), nitrogen oxides, particulate matter, volatile organic compounds, cigarette smoke, arsenic and heavy metals?

When we expose ourselves to pollution for a prolonged period of time or repeatedly, the fighter antioxidants such as vitamin C, vitamin E, superoxide dismutase and glutathione reductase get depleted from the skin. This results in the production of more free radicals and reactive oxygen species which are the villains that damage the DNA of the skin and disrupt the skin's barrier function.

This can lead to dryness, discolouration, fine lines and wrinkles. Long-term exposure to air pollution can also cause skin allergies, eczema and even acne.

PAH are formed in any burning, waste incineration, metal production, fuel and wood combustion. Exposure to PAH can result in acne-like eruptions on the face, chest and back. PAHs have also been implicated in the development of skin cancer.[*]

Particulate matter in the air consists of mixtures of various sizes and compositions from factories, power plants, refuse incinerators, automobiles, construction activities, fires and natural windblown dust.[†] What is

---

[*] A.O. Fernandez and A. Banerji, 'Inhibition of Benzopyrene Induced for Stomach Tumors by Field Bean Protease Inhibitors(s)', *Carcinogenesis* 16 (1995): 1843–46.

[†] U. Pöschl. 'Atmospheric Aerosols: Composition, Transformation, Climate and Health Effects', *Angewandte Chemie International Edition in English* 44, no. 46 (2005): 7520–40.

more appalling is that the most harmful components of particulate matter are nanosized particles from traffic pollution.

Particulate matter penetrates the skin either through hair follicles or through the skin's pores and exerts its detrimental effects, contributing to skin ageing, pigment spots, wrinkles, lax skin and spider veins.[*]

A study published in the *Journal of Investigative Dermatology* showed that increase in soot and particles from traffic was associated with 20 per cent more pigment spots on the forehead and cheeks.[†]

Further, a study in Korea has shown that symptoms of atopic eczema increases in children who have shifted to a new building due to an increase in exposure to volatile organic compounds.[‡]

Closer home, you will be surprised to know that there are 1.3 million deaths in India each year due to poor indoor air quality. The most common reason for indoor pollution is the use of firewood, cow dung cake, coal, charcoal, kerosene for cooking. Among the 70 per cent of the country's rural population, about 80 per cent of households rely on biomass fuel, making India top the list of countries with the largest population lacking access to

[*] A. Vierkötter et al., 'Airborne Particle Exposure and Extrinsic Skin Ageing', *Journal of Investigative Dermatology* 130 (2010): 2719–26; N.L. Mills et al., 'Combustion-derived Nanoparticulate Induces the Adverse Vascular Effects of Diesel Exhaust Inhalation', *European Heart Journal* 32 (2011): 2660–71.
[†] A. Vierkötter et al., 'Airborne Particle Exposure and Extrinsic Skin Aging', *Journal of Investigative Dermatology* 130 (2010): 2719–26.
[‡] R. Dales et al., 'Quality of Indoor Residential Air and Health', *Canadian Medical Association Journal* 179 (2008): 147–52.

cleaner fuel for cooking. Tobacco smoke, organic solvents in paints and varnishes and exhaust from cars in the garage are some of the other causes for indoor pollution.*

Skincare and protection from pollution

Always cleanse your skin well after returning from any outdoor place. Use a facewash which can unclog your pores and remove all the dirt and grime from the skin's surface as well as the pollutant particles which sit on the skin.

Next, make sure you apply a good moisturizer. Pollution dehydrates the skin, leaving it dull and more exposed to environmental damage. A moisturizer will protect the lipid barrier layer of the skin.

Do not forget to apply a sunscreen with both UVA and UVB protection. Choose physical sunblocks which will also form a protective layer on the skin, making it difficult for the smog particles to reach the deeper layers of the skin.

At night, make sure you apply a serum or cream containing vitamin C and E, which will detox your skin.

Do not forget to wear a mask which not only covers your nose and mouth but also your entire face except the eyes. Physical protection is the best method of protection from pollutant particles. This is extremely important for people with high occupational risk, such as traffic policemen and sweepers.

---

* E.H. Kim et al., 'Indoor Air Pollution Aggravates Symptoms of Atopic Dermatitis in Children', *PLOS One* 10, no. 3 (2015).

Make sure you drink enough water, a minimum of two litres every day, and have a lot of bright-coloured fruits such as berries, pomegranates and dark grapes that are rich in antioxidants.

You may also take vitamin C, E and A supplements to protect the skin. Supplements of polypodium leucotomos, a potent antioxidant, prevents cellular damage from exposure to harmful rays.

In extreme conditions, you must have an air purifier at home so that at least in your safe haven you are breathing clean air.

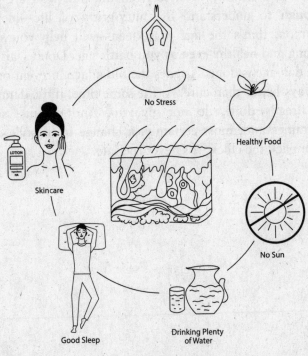

Good lifestyle

Aye	Nay
Cleanse	Sleep with make-up on
Moisturize	Smoking
Sunscreen	Alcohol
Make-up removal	Pollution
Sleep	Late nights
Healthy food	Junk food, sugar
Exercise	Lazing
Meditate	Stress

Leading a healthy lifestyle from the time you are old enough to understand the nitty-gritty of life—in my opinion, that's the age of sixteen—will help you stay young and healthy even as you battle age. Don't wait till the damage is done. As goes the old adage, prevention is always better than cure. At the same time, if the damage is already done, do not give up. Antioxidants, skin therapies and, most certainly, a change in lifestyle can turn back the clock. It's never too late.

WEEK 6

16

When Should You See a Dermat?

'Three things are needed for success in painting and sculpture: to see beauty when young and accustom oneself to it, to work hard, and to obtain good advice'
—Bernini

'Doc, I never had pigmentation issues earlier and my skin was flawless,' said Mickey's forty-one-year-old cousin Sheela, whom Mickey had dragged to my clinic after seeing the changes in her own skin. 'My lifestyle is the same. My diet hasn't changed. But now, I see these dark patches on my face suddenly. And people even tell me that I have started to look tired and old.' Sheela was an athlete in college. Running was her passion, whether in the hot summers or cold winters. She never used a sunscreen because it would get washed out with her sweat. After marriage, she quit sports but led a hectic life. I explained to Sheela that the damage was inflicted during her teens and twenties when she ran in the sun for hours together, had no set pattern for food or sleep and barely got time to relax. The effects start showing only in our late thirties and forties. With age, the ability of our skin cells to repair themselves slow down. This makes things worse and problems such as pigmentation, adult acne, sagging skin, wrinkles and eczemas start manifesting. It is better to start skincare early, in your teens, and see a dermatologist in order to understand you skin.

My patient Vivian used to play cricket for his college but now works indoors in a bank. When he came to consult me, he said he had given up on sunscreens. He had tried every sunscreen available in the shops because he thought he was getting permanently tanned—he had developed sun-induced pigmentation on the face. After examining him, I gave him a water-based sunscreen which did not leave his skin white. Additionally, I also gave him a three-month sunscreen challenge to make him believe in the benefits of using one. Fortunately, he was sporting and obedient enough to take up the challenge. And in three months, he saw his skin looking clearer and vowed never to forget to apply a sunscreen on all the exposed parts of his body before stepping out. Had Vivian consulted a dermatologist right at the beginning, his tryst with sunscreens wouldn't have begun in the first place. In my opinion, one should meet a dermatologist once you hit sixteen and again at thirty and at forty-five. Your skin changes according to age, hormones, lifestyle, climate and pollution, and only a dermatologist can help you with the correct skincare routine.

There are a myriad creams and lotions available to the consumer in the market, making it tough for a person to choose the right product for himself or herself. Hence a visit to a dermatologist becomes important. One also needs to see a dermatologist for certain skin conditions which may not seem severe but don't seem to abate despite efforts. For instance, severe acne or pimples will not improve with over-the-counter products. If after a month of using an anti-acne cream you still see no results, it is time to see a dermatologist. You may be suffering from hormonal imbalances or PCOS. Similarly, if you have developed scars or blemishes, you should not try out treatments on your own. Let your dermatologist do the peels and lasers suitable for you.

If you see a mole or an abnormal growth on your skin which keeps growing, you must seek help. The mole could be turning cancerous or the growth could be an infected cyst.

Eczema, psoriasis and other types of dermatitis are accompanied by itching and rashes. They may subside temporarily with an over-the-counter steroid cream or an anti-allergic pill but will only worsen once you stop the medication. Make sure you consult a dermatologist for any rashes on your body.

Dandruff—a common problem—may also need a dermatologist's attention. If you have used all kinds of anti-dandruff shampoos with no results, and tried all anti-dandruff treatments in salons, it could be possible that your problem is something else altogether. For all you know, you may be suffering from scalp disorders such as seborrhoeic dermatitis or psoriasis which mimic dandruff but are seen as thicker, stickier scales on the scalp. They need medical attention. Scar-reduction creams may help if the scars are superficial. However, if they are raised, thickened scars or keloids, you must consult a dermatologist as you may need injections into the keloid or cryotherapy with liquid nitrogen. Similarly for depressed scars, you may need fractional laser treatment. So don't just rely on microdermabrasions and other treatments at your local beauty parlour.

Brown skin discolouration and pigmentation reduce with over-the-counter skin-lightening creams. However, the pigmentation returns when you stop using these creams. Sometimes, long-term use of these creams causes thinning of the skin, visible veins and sensitive skin due to a steroid present in the cream. Other times they can cause more pigmentation due to the presence of hydroquinone in the cream. Hence, do not try over-the-counter skin lighteners.

And of course, if you have an important occasion like Mickey's, you must consult a dermatologist at least six weeks in advance. If you have skin problems like severe acne, pigmentation, etc., then you need to see the dermatologist not six weeks, but six months in advance. Having said that, don't panic if you don't have six months. We dermatologists always have quick fixes for you.

17

Skin Treatments

'The true work of art is but a shadow of the divine perfection'

—Michelangelo

Mickey had a few days left and I had to do some behind-the-scenes magic to make her skin even-toned, more radiant and blemish-free. Sometimes creams may not be enough for certain skin problems such as acne scars, pigmentation, sagging skin and wrinkles. At other times, you may need to spruce yourself up for an important event. There are various skin treatments available to aid this pursuit. When you read about them in the newspapers or online, be careful not to trip up. Let us discuss some of them:

- Skin polishing
- Chemical peel
- Microneedling
- Mesotherapy
- Lasers

- Radio frequency skin tightening
- High-intensity focused ultrasound (HIFU)
- Threads
- Platelet-rich plasma
- Botox
- Fillers
- Skin boosters

Skin polishing

A lot of people come a day before an event, a party or a wedding wanting to get their skin polished in the hope that their pigmentation will disappear like magic. Let me debunk this myth. Skin polishing is a more sophisticated way of exfoliating your skin. It is done with a vacuum-operated device which sucks all the dead skin and grime from the pores. It also has fine aluminium oxide crystals or fine diamond powder which exfoliates the skin gently. This is an excellent way to cleanse the skin but do not go for it more than once a month if you have dry skin and once in fifteen days if you have oily skin. Skin polishing helps remove tan and very superficial acne marks. However, one session is never enough. One has to get about four to six sessions done to get optimum results. The good thing is, after the session, one comes out feeling cleaner. It does not have any side effects and is a lunchtime procedure. So you can walk back to your office without anyone asking you any weird questions. You may certainly get compliments like, 'Whoa, you look fresh!' 'I realize that regular clean-ups at a qualified dermatologist's clinic are better than facials at your neighbourhood parlour,' says actor Richa Chadha.

Chemical peel

The moment I suggest a chemical peel to my patient, the answer is always, 'No, doc, I do not want to apply chemicals on my face.'

The truth is any cream or lotion that you apply on the face may have the same chemicals that you apply as a peel—the difference being, the peel will have a higher concentration. Most of the times, these so-called chemical peels are extracts of fruits, tree barks, seeds or leaves. They are called 'chemical' because of their chemical formula and the preservatives added to the peel solution. You will understand better when you look at the sources of most of the chemical peels. Glycolic acid, for example, is an extract of sugar cane, lactic acid is a milk extract, mandelic acid is derived from bitter almonds and kojic acid from Japanese mushrooms, salicylic acid from willow bark.

'Doc, I cannot do a peel. Lying down on a treatment bed for an hour is just not my thing,' said Sandeep, a patient. Who said it will take an hour? You walk in, your face is cleansed and degreased. The peel solution is applied for five to ten minutes and then removed. A sunscreen is applied and you are ready to go back to work. Some peels are cream-based; they are applied to the skin and left on for four to eight hours. So it is the quickest skin treatment you can think of.

Miraya had been refraining from doing a peel for a long time because she saw her friend shed skin like a snake after having done a peel. Well, chemical peels are classified as superficial, medium and deep, based on how deep into the skin the peel solution penetrates. Medium peel solutions cause peeling of skin for three to four days. They are usually done for acne blemishes, pigmentation, fine lines, open pores and even pimples. Deep peels cause peeling for up to ten days but are not recommended for Indian skin. Superficial peels do not cause visible skin peeling. And they work wonders when it comes to radiance and glow.

'Doc, I have heard skin becomes sensitive after doing a peel,' said Ruhi, another of my patients. Choosing the right peel for your skin along with proper post-peel care will certainly never make your skin sensitive.

A word of advice: Make sure you do not step out in the sun after a peel. Also, some peels such as TCA, retinol and phenol cause peeling of the skin. Let this happen naturally. Do not try to remove the skin which looks like snake skin, however tempted you may be.

Microneedling

Microneedling is a procedure whereby tiny channels are created in the skin with very fine medical-grade stainless steel needles, which are either fixed on a roller or a pen-like device. 'I read that microneedling is popular with celebrities like Jennifer Aniston, Kim Kardashian, Angelina Jolie, Brad Pitt and Demi Moore. May I also do microneedling for my face?' asked thirty-year-old Ashwin, who was troubled with the pits on his face that pimples had left behind. He wanted to be an actor but the tiny scars on his face were acting like speed breakers to his confidence. Yes, Ashwin could do microneedling along with a couple of other treatments to get rid of his acne scars. Microneedling is also done to reduce pores, stretch marks, accident scars and also to get radiant skin.

The instrument used for microneedling is called dermaroller or dermapen. A dermaroller is a plastic handheld device with a drum-shaped head which has 192 needles all around it. These needles are 0.5–3 mm long. A dermapen is a motorized device with similar needles attached to a pen-like structure. The patient's skin is cleansed and a numbing cream is applied for about an hour. The skin is cleaned with sterile aseptic solutions. The roller is then rolled on the skin in four directions. The skin is cleaned and a vitamin C serum or hyaluronic acid is applied on it. The patient is then sent home. The procedure feels like a sting but is bearable. The redness and swelling persists for a day or two at the most. The skin looks radiant and taut after microneedling. Acne scars reduce over a period of time. The dermatologist decides on the type of roller, i.e. the number of needles and their length, depending on the condition and area to be treated. For example, a 0.5 mm needle length is used for the under-eye area because the skin here is very thin. For the treatment of acne scars, 2 mm needles are required.

Mesotherapy

Actress Jennifer Aniston and singer Katy Perry have endorsed this celebrity trend of injecting minerals and vitamins directly into the skin in order to nourish it and make it more youthful. One of my celebrity clients says that it reduces blotchiness, makes the skin look young, soft and radiant. Mesotherapy involves infusing vitamins,

minerals, amino acids, enzymes and hyaluronic acid into
the mesoderm, i.e. the middle layer of the skin, either with
a dermaroller or a mesogun or even micro-injections,
directly into the skin. It is painless and often qualifies as
a lunchtime facial. It is done once in two weeks for six to
eight sessions. The discomfort is bearable, akin to having
your arms waxed.

Lasers

Talk about lasers and some of my patients want to
scoot from my clinic like I have asked them to commit
suicide! But you will certainly regret it if you get a laser
treatment done from a person who doesn't have sound
knowledge of the device but has enough money to buy
the machine. The word LASER is an acronym for 'light
amplification by stimulated emission of radiation'. When
we say radiation, it is not the radiation energy which
can harm your DNA or your cells. Some people ask me
if laser can damage internal organs. Well, laser energy
can only penetrate up to a certain layer in the skin and
not beneath. So there is no question of harming internal
organs. The only part of the body which can get affected
is the eye. Hence, one must use protective eye shields
before performing any such treatment.

When Abimanyu came to me with a lot of stubborn
pigmentation on his forehead, I suggested doing a laser
treatment. 'But I don't want my hair gone, doc,' he said.
Well, laser treatment doesn't just involve hair removal. There
are several types of laser with specific wavelengths and they
can be used for different treatments. A long pulse diode or

a long pulse Nd Yag, an Alexandrite laser are excellent for removing hair on skin like ours, the Indian skin.

'Doc, tell me some other method to get rid of my hair. My friend has done twenty sessions of laser hair removal and it's still growing back long,' said one of my patients, Pritika.

Hair regrowth can happen if you have a hormonal imbalance in the body. Usually, a female needs eight to ten sessions of laser to get rid of the hair and a male needs twelve to fifteen. But if a girl has polycystic ovaries, raised prolactin levels or raised androgen levels, or even insulin resistance, her response to laser will be extremely slow and the laser sessions may go on and on. Similarly, if the guy is taking supplements such as anabolic steroids or growth hormones or similar stuff, his response to laser will be very slow or even zero. So one must get all hormones checked before going for laser hair removal. Get the hormonal imbalance treated, lose weight and then expect fabulous results. Otherwise be prepared to do multiple laser sessions.

A Q-switched Nd Yag laser is used to remove tattoos, reduce pigmentation, cause skin brightening. It is also used to remove certain types of birthmarks and even reduce freckles.

Resurfacing lasers such as Fractional CO_2 or fractional erbium lasers are used to treat scars or depressions which occur after acne, accident scars, scars which remain after burns or surgeries. They are also used to reduce fine lines, open pores and stretch marks.

Pulsed dye lasers are used to get rid of those spider veins or thin pink veins which are visible through the skin. They are also used to treat bigger problems like blood vessel malformations since birth.

Indian skin tends to pigment during the healing process after undergoing any peel, laser or even surgery, if one does not take proper care after the treatment. This pigmentation, known as post-inflammatory hyperpigmentation is indeed temporary but can be bothersome and stay for up to six to eight months. So it is better to take some basic pre- and post-treatment precautions.

Whichever laser you do, you must avoid direct sun exposure for at least seventy-two hours after the treatment. Avoid using scrubs or swimming, bleaching, body scrubs, massages for at least a week after a laser.

Radio frequency and HIFU

'Dr J, I want to look ten years younger but I do not want to go under the knife,' said fifty-six-year-old Manjula. Had Manjula said this to me twenty years ago, I would have had little to offer her. But today, technology has given us fabulous anti-ageing weapons which are harmless and efficacious.

Non-surgical skin tightening can be done using radio frequency energy or high-intensity focused ultrasound. Both technologies are used to tighten collagen fibres which tend to loosen and wither with age or even poor lifestyle. Both treatments involve passing heat energy to the dermis of the skin which is home to collagen and elastin fibres. This heat energy tightens collagen and elastin and also stimulates new collagen formation over three to four months. Now, only a dermatologist can decide whether your skin will respond to radio frequency or HIFU. So if you want to treat irritating jowls, wrinkles and folds on the face and saggy skin on the face and body, consult your dermatologist without fearing to go under the knife. While radio frequency skin tightening will have you walk out of the clinic as if nothing has happened, with HIFU, be prepared to be a little swollen for four to five days after the treatment. Since there is no light energy involved, there are no chances of burns or pigmentation after treatment. Hence, these treatments are extremely safe. These treatments may not show very satisfactory results in people who are very chubby, hence lose a little fat and then go for tightening procedures.

Thread lifts

'Doc, you've got to be kidding. Threads into the face? Are you going to sew my face with a needle and thread?' asked forty-eight-year-old Meher when I suggested a thread lift as the best option for her sagging face. Meher has a lean and pretty face but her jowls are now prominent. The chiselled jawline she once flaunted is now like a small hill-and-valley. It bothers her the most. She had consulted a plastic surgeon who advised a facelift surgery. But she wasn't ready to go under the knife yet. She had decided to undergo a facelift as a sixtieth birthday gift to herself. She did not want to battle a sagging jaw for twelve more years and that is when someone recommended her to me.

Thread lift is an office procedure where the thread is inserted into the skin along vectors to tighten the skin, be it in the jowls or neck or even cheeks and forehead.

The two types of threads commonly used are polydioxanone threads and silhouette threads.

These are fine threads which are inserted into the skin after applying a numbing cream. They stimulate new collagen formation within two to three months of inserting them in the right plane, and this helps tighten the skin. The threads dissolve over three to four months. In this, two sessions are usually done at an interval of one month. Thereafter the procedure needs to be repeated after a year. If you are in your late forties or fifties and have loose skin under your chin, a sagging jawline or if you feel your cheeks are sagging, this could be a good option for you. There is a little swelling on the face for three to four days after the treatment. However, there are no other side effects. You can walk into the clinic, get your treatment done and walk back to work after two hours.

Platelet-rich plasma (PRP) or the vampire facial

Kim Kardashian made headlines when she posted a video of herself getting PRP injections all over her face way back in 2013. She called it the vampire facial, not because it would be done at night (it is pretty much done during the day) but because it is bloody and looks gory. The process involves collecting one's own blood, putting it through an incubator followed by a centrifuge to draw out plasma rich in platelets and growth factors. This plasma is reinjected into the skin of the same person, on the face, neck, hands or whichever part of the body that needs to be treated. Treated for what? Well, for fine lines, wrinkles, dullness, large pores, blotchy skin, acne scars or even stretch marks that you hate. It is done in all age groups from twenty to sixty and is absolutely safe. Bruising may be the only side effect but this too is temporary and lasts for four to five days.

The latest trend is to do a round of microneedling and then just pour the PRP on the skin surface which has many channels opened up due to the microneedling. We also add hyaluronic acid to the PRP for more hydration and better stimulation of fibroblasts, cells which produce collagen.

Botulinum toxin (Botox)

'Doc, I watched myself on Instagram stories today and I could see one thousand lines on my face. And it makes me look old,' said Abigail, a thirty-seven-year-old home-maker. These lines and wrinkles on the face which come with emoting are expression lines. They occur due to constant movement of the muscles as our face emotes a thousand different expressions. Every time we laugh, cry, talk, worry, get angry, look surprised or feel sad, the muscles, the fat above the muscle and skin move in particular directions. Over time, this constant movement results in wrinkles or lines. 'Abigail, you must be a very expressive person, but don't worry. It is good to let your face speak,' I told her. Since she was thirty-seven, and the lines were bothering her so much, I decided to soften a few lines. I told her I would inject a few units of Botox to get rid of her crow's feet around the eyes and reduce the frown lines between her eyebrows. I would then do some hyaluronic acid filler injections to reduce her laugh lines.

Just as the word Xerox is used for photocopy, a neuromodulator injection comprising of botulinum toxin has become synonymous with the word Botox. Botox is a natural, purified protein available in the form of an injection. Upon injecting into the muscle, it relaxes the wrinkle-causing muscles and creates a rejuvenated and youthful appearance. It is US FDA approved, well researched and safe to use.

Let's understand the uses of Botox. Botox is used to soften or erase:

- Frown lines between the eyebrows
- Crow's feet around the eyes
- Forehead wrinkles
- Bunny lines on the nose
- Downturned corners of the lips (sad lips)
- Neck bands also known as turkey neck
- Horizontal lines on neck
- Multiple dimples on the chin
- Square jaw
- Excessive sweating of underarms, palms and feet

Shubha, forty-seven years old, yearned for a good jawline. Her neck looked like that of a turkey and she hated it. So I injected a few units of Botox into her neck and jawline to erase the neck bands and create a nice jawline. This procedure is also called the Nefertiti lift, named after the beautiful Egyptian queen Nefertiti. I usually recommend Botox for people above thirty-five years of age and only if necessary. The results are seen within three or four days but the effect is best seen after seven to fifteen days of injection. The effects gradually wear off after four to six months and the treatment has to be repeated. People who are above twenty-five years of age and have a very broad jaw or a square face due to strong masseter muscle (the muscle used for chewing) can take Botox injections to reduce the size of the jaw and make it more oval or rounded. I wouldn't recommend cosmetic Botox for other indications in youngsters. Botox is also given to reduce excessive sweating on palms and underarms, and for the treatment of migraine.

A word of caution: If the doctor who is injecting isn't well-trained, mistakes may happen. So make sure you go to a qualified and well-trained dermatologist or plastic surgeon. Do not get obsessed and go overboard with Botox. Too much can lead to loss of expression lines and give you a plastic face. The aim should be to soften the lines and look natural.

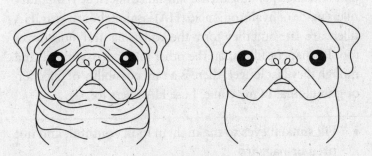

Overdose of Botox

Botox is manufactured by Allergan. Other botulinum toxin injections available are Xeomin and Dysport, both of which are also US FDA approved.

Fillers

Like I mentioned in chapter 11, as we age, the skin loses its collagen and elastin fibres, the fat below the skin gets displaced from some places and lost from the others. The muscles become weaker. The deeper pockets of fat are lost and the bone shrinks too. All these changes happen gradually, leading to the formation of laugh lines, jowls, sunken eyes, thinner lips, retruded chin and even hollow temples. The skin support system undergoes a failure and the pillars need to be recreated to give the face its support. This is done with the help of filler injections. Fillers are not the same as Botox. They do not have any effect on expression lines or wrinkles.

Fillers are available as pre-filled injections which are injected into the skin into all the hollow areas of the face to recreate the youthfulness. They may be temporary or permanent, depending on the substance injected. Temporary fillers made of hyaluronic acid (HA) last for about a year. HA fillers are safe and they form the body's natural moisturizer too. Permanent fillers, on the other hand, are synthetic and though they last longer, there is a rare possibility of infection or granuloma. In my clinic, I use HA fillers to:

- Fill sunken eyes to make them look youthful, and not tired or haggard
- Fill brows to lift them

- Fill the temples, which become hollow with age
- Fill the cheeks, which become flat with age
- Recreate cheekbones in younger women
- Create a sharper nose without surgery
- Fill thin lips or create a subtle pout in order to make one look attractive. Lips can be filled beautifully without making them look huge and artificial. The key is to keep it natural and not have the lips walk into a room before the person herself.
- Make laugh lines less prominent
- Recreate a sharp jawline
- Create a nice chin in those with small chins. This improves the contour of the face.
- Fill thin earlobes so that earrings can be worn without the lobe sagging down
- Fill hands which look wrinkled and old

Why do I consider it better than surgery?

- It's cheaper.
- If one doesn't like the way the face looks after the injection, it can be dissolved with another injection called hyaluronidase within two hours. So you don't live with it for life.
- You don't have to go under the knife.
- Lunchtime procedure, no hospitalization.
- No anaesthesia given. Just ice or a topical anaesthetic cream applied.
- No downtime or recovery period, you can go back to work immediately.
- Safer as there is no risk of surgical complications.

- Results are seen instantly, as opposed to a surgery where it takes six to ten months.

I love to inject fillers to bring back the youthfulness in a male or female face. I inject fillers to recreate the emotions of joy. I inject fillers to instil confidence in the person by getting rid of those tired eyes and hollow cheeks. I inject fillers to enhance one's facial features to make them more attractive, not overdone. I inject fillers to improve the overall facial contour to replicate one's youth and not make a person look like someone else. It is a combination of a lot of study of the human anatomy coupled with the art of sculpting a beautiful face. The key lies in the art of injecting the right way and having an eye for natural beauty.

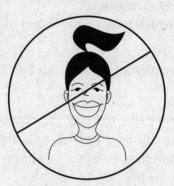

Overdone lip filler injection

Skin boosters

The skin is injected with tiny doses of hyaluronic acid, a natural constituent of the skin lost with ageing. Hyaluronic acid has a property of binding and holding water in the skin. Hence it improves skin hydration, giving a glowing complexion by naturally smoothening the skin from within. In this, multiple tiny injections are given to the skin after numbing it with a cream, thereby reducing the discomfort. Injections are spaced at three to four weeks for three sessions and repeat sessions are needed no earlier than six months. With just three sessions, the skin looks and feels supple and radiant. These injections are available as Belotero Hydro and Restylane Vital in India.

There is no one-size-fits-all when it comes to aesthetic treatments. Every individual has unique skin with different requirements. Treatments have to be mixed and matched according to the need of the individual. As I mentioned earlier, one may need a combination of chemical peels, laser resurfacing and microneedling to reduce deep scars which are formed due to acne. Similarly, to make the face look tighter and younger, one may have to undergo a combination of radio frequency tightening and HIFU, and sometimes fillers and Botox injections too. You must also remember to follow your skincare ritual along with these treatments for better results. Furthermore, none of these procedures are permanent. So have realistic expectations and take care of your skin every single day. Consistence is the key to beautiful skin.

I did one yellow peel and one session of laser toning for Mickey. I also scheduled a photo-facial for her a week before her wedding to give her skin that final zing.

18

Latest Advancements in Skin Technology

'Some painters transform the sun into a yellow spot,
others transform a yellow spot into the sun'
—Pablo Picasso

When it comes to skin and beauty, technology is advancing at a rocket speed. A lot of research has been going on in the field of cosmetic dermatology and aesthetic medicine. A number of people are now keen on non-invasive cosmetic procedures to look better and younger. With a few game-changing innovations, one can now have clearer, tighter and more radiant skin. Not only that, the body can be brought back to shape without having to go under the knife. The American Society of Plastic Surgeons revealed that 15.7 million non-invasive cosmetic dermatology procedures were performed in the United States in the year 2017. Non-invasive fat-reducing procedures using CoolSculpt increased by 7 per cent, non-invasive cellulite treatment increased by 19 per cent and non-surgical skin-tightening treatments increased by 9 per cent. So the market is booming and people are certainly getting more aware of their skin and body.

Let me throw some light on some of the *happening* treatments and regimes.

CoolSculpting

CoolSculpting is the hottest trend in Hollywood right now and India is not far behind.

While Kris Kardashian was seen undergoing CoolSculpting in the television series *Keeping up with the Kardashians*, Khloe Kardashian has spoken about it on her social media accounts. American model and actress Molly Sims shared her CoolSculpting experience with a popular magazine, saying that it helped her get rid of her unwanted, stubborn belly fat post pregnancy.

Over 6 million CoolSculpting treatments have been done all over the world with successful outcomes. And these people are not just celebrities; they are people like you and me who want to look good and feel confident without having to be concerned about the abnormal bulges on their body. CoolSculpting is the only US FDA–approved treatment for non-surgical fat reduction. One does not have to be hospitalized or given anaesthesia, and there are no cuts and stitches on your body. You can walk out of the clinic comfortably on your own once your treatment gets over. CoolSculpting uses cryolipolysis technology to destroy fat cells which lie beneath the skin. The procedure freezes fat cells and destroys them. These fat cells get eliminated from the body over the next eight to twelve weeks. The device used in the treatment has an in-built safety mechanism that ensures no harm is done to the skin above the fat. A muffin top, the ugly underarm puff, love handles, back fat, little bulges on the thigh—not much, but just enough to show through a snug-fitting T-shirt or blouse or jeans—can be made to disappear with cryolipolysis. Remember, CoolSculpting is not a weight-loss treatment. It's for people who are healthy but have bulges that refuse to budge, no matter how healthy a diet they follow or how many kilometres they run or swim. Your BMI should be between 20 and 30 if you want to go for CoolSculpting. If you are obese or even moderately overweight with BMI above 30, please do not consider this treatment.

Armanda, my thirty-four-year-old manager, told me one day that no matter how healthy she ate or how regularly she exercised, she always had a few areas on her body where the fat just wouldn't budge. She had developed these bulges after her pregnancy. I asked her to undergo liposuction but she was afraid of surgery. 'Besides, I am no model or actress, doc,' she said. Nonetheless, these stubborn love handles and back fat bothered her all the time. She yearned to wear a perfectly fitted dress someday but was afraid her bulges would show. Finally, CoolSculpting came to her rescue.

At my clinic, we use the CoolSculpting machine by Allergan, the original cryolipolysis device approved by

US FDA. It has a paddle-like applicator attached to a hose that provides the cold. Applicators come in various sizes to suit the area to be treated. For example, the cool mini applicator is meant for the double chin, the cool advantage applicator is meant for love handles and so on. This applicator securely pulls up the area to be treated between its two panels and the fat cells crystallized for about forty-five minutes. You may feel a slight stinging or a sensation of cramping once the treatment is complete. You may also see a temporary whitening or reddening of the treated area, which may also feel stiff. Otherwise, you're free to resume normal activity immediately after the treatment. Men and women can both opt for the treatment. In fact, many men are now looking at ripped bodies and go regularly to the gym. They still have some stubborn bulges. We help them get rid of these bulges with this treatment.

For many, a single session is enough to produce great results, provided you keep your expectations realistic. On an average, most patients see 20–30 per cent fat reduction. That may not sound like a lot, but visually it can mean the difference between a flat stomach and a paunch.

The most common side effects, all of which are typically resolved within one to three weeks, are redness, swelling and bruising. Cryolipolysis with CoolSculpt does not harm the skin or muscle tissue; rather, the cold temperature specifically targets fat cells. What you need to keep in mind is that for any treatment to sustain, maintenance is the key. So make sure you keep a check on your diet and don't go binging once you have lost those bulges. Exercising for at least half an hour every day would do you wonders.

Fat lipolysis injections

'Can you melt my double chin away? I always have to try different angles to make sure my double chin doesn't make me look like a toad in my selfies,' said Ivana, who hated her double chin. Ivana did not have a big double chin. So I did not suggest CoolSculpting which would have been otherwise great. There was a small lump of fat and I knew the easy way out. It's called Kybella or Geolysis. This is a US FDA–approved injection containing sodium deoxycholate which is injected carefully into the fat layer. It actually breaks down the fat cells which are then excreted through the lymphatics. The downside is, there is visual swelling in the area of injection for five to seven days. It does subside and the chin looks like it was always flat and well shaped. For larger pockets of fat under the skin, I would suggest the CoolMini cryolipolysis. It just works like magic in a single session.

Micro-Botox

In this, Botox is diluted ten times and tiny droplets are injected into the superficial skin instead of the muscle. Micro-Botox reduces oiliness, closes pore size and makes the skin appear taut. It is given once in three to four months all over the face and neck. It also gives a nice sheen to the face. Women who are tired of crinkled neck, micro-Botox is for you. There are no precautions for micro-Botox injections as they are really miniscule doses.

Non-surgical nose jobs

'Really? Can my nose look sharper without getting a nose job done?' Anupriya was gorgeous but always complained about her nose being flat. It bothered her especially when she had to face the camera. But she wasn't allowed to undergo any surgery. 'Anything non-surgical, doc,' said her mom. So I decided to give her filler injections to create a sharper nose. HA filler injections are given into the nasal bridge to create a well-defined, sharp nose. The effect lasts for up to two years. Non-surgical nose jobs can't make the nose smaller, but they can help correct imperfections and camouflage areas that are bothersome. Anupriya loved her nose job. She didn't have to take leave from work nor did she have to worry about swelling, pain and bruising, and most importantly, no one could tell. But almost everyone who saw her commented on how beautiful she looked.

Filler injections for the body

Aunty Akshara looked gorgeous at fifty-eight. It was her thirty-fifth wedding anniversary, and she had worn a bright red Kanjeevaram silk saree, flowers adorning her hair, which was tied in a bun. She was bedecked from head to toe but her ears were bare. Her earlobes had thinned with age, and to top it, the hefty earrings she routinely wore dragged her earlobes down. I also noticed her hands. They looked shrivelled and wrinkled like a dry raisin. I asked her to see me at the clinic. 'I am going to give you the best anniversary gift,' I whispered into her ears as I left the party.

She was promptly there at my clinic at 10 a.m. the next day. She knew I do not make false promises. I told her my aesthetic-dermatology eyes noticed her ears and hands at the party and I certainly didn't want my precious aunt to have any telltale signs of ageing. I applied a numbing cream on her earlobes and hands and gave her some magazines to read as she sat with the cream on her skin for forty-five minutes. Then, I plumped her earlobes by injecting HA fillers. I also injected calcium hydroxyapatite–based fillers into the top layer of her skin on the hands. Her earlobes were ready to bear the brunt of her earrings again and her hands looked smooth as that of a twenty-year-old. She was thrilled beyond words. Fillers made of hyaluronic acid, calcium hydroxyapatite, poly lactic acid and poly methyl methacrylate are now being used to fill thin earlobes, wrinkled hands and feet. Koreans like fuller calves and Brazilians love big butts. So fillers are even being injected into calves, buttocks and breasts. It is always safer to use temporary HA fillers or semi-permanent fillers such as Radiesse made of calcium hydroxyapatite and Scupltra made of poly L-lactic acid. Avoid permanent fillers as there may be chances of infection, granulomas or disfigurement over the years.

Vaginal skin tightening

This is not something to shy away from. After childbirth and with age, the lips of the vagina do get thin and lax. HA fillers can be used to reshape the lips. Vaginal skin tightening can also be done using radio frequency skin tightening devices and lasers. The treatment is similar to the radio frequency treatments described in chapter 17. Always opt for US FDA–approved devices only. Also make sure you go to really hygienic and reputed clinics.

Cellfina

'Doc, do something about these dimples on my thighs. My entire butt and thighs look like hills and valleys,' said Niharika, my twenty-nine-year-old patient. She had tried all possible creams which claimed they were the miracle cures for cellulite but nothing worked. Cellulite occurs when swollen fat cells get trapped in the skin and the lymphatic drainage is impaired. It is seen in both slim and obese females and becomes more prominent with age. The condition has been extremely difficult to treat in spite of diets, loss of weight, exercise and even skin-tightening or fat-reduction procedures.

Cellfina is a US FDA–approved breakthrough treatment which can actually improve the appearance of cellulite. A needle-sized device is used to break the fibrous bands amid which the fat cells are trapped. This evens out the fat cells and smoothens the dimpling. Results are seen in a week and last for up to three years. Though the treatment is done using local anaesthesia, it is done as an office procedure.

Cryotherapy

Cryotherapy has been around for decades at dermatology clinics for the treatment of warts, acne scars, skin growths and even skin cancer. But it is being propagated for anti-ageing in recent years and is popularly known as Frotox. In this procedure, liquid nitrogen is sprayed on the skin's surface. The freezing of the skin causes constriction of blood vessels, thereby reducing flushing, redness and inflammation. It also causes mild exfoliation and helps in reducing acne as well as superficial acne scars. It stimulates collagen formation which leads to tightening of the skin. There are full-body cryo chambers where a person exposes the entire body to the freezing liquid nitrogen, which has a temperature of about -90° C, for two to four minutes. The extreme cold stimulates new collagen synthesis and reduces inflammation in the cells. While the long-term effects are skin tightening, the bonus is an instant glow. This is because the extreme cold causes blood vessels to constrict, and when you step out, they open up again. So the blood gushes back to the skin, making it flush with radiance.

LED

Scroll through Instagram pictures of Hollywood celebrities and you will find most of them wearing these well-lit ghostlike masks. No, they are not celebrating Halloween. These are LED masks which may have blue or red light. LED stands for 'light-emitting diode'. If your blackheads and whiteheads are turning into a menace, use a blue light to kill the bacteria which cause acne. And if you want your skin to look firm and pores invisible, red LED is the right choice for you. Red light speeds up healing and stimulates collagen production and is a perfect ten-minute anti-ageing facial. Results are temporary. However, you will see results after four to five sessions. It is painless, non-invasive and there are no telltale signs.

Stem cell injections

After the vampire facial, this is going to be the next big thing. It is still undergoing a lot of research and does not have US FDA clearance yet, but a lot of clinics in Europe boast of doing stem cell therapy for anti-ageing. In this, adipose tissue or fat cells are removed from the person's abdomen or buttocks. These fats cells are sent to a laboratory where stem cells are obtained from the fat cells. These stem cells are then injected into the face to create a youthful, wrinkle-free face. Stem cells are also obtained from the bone marrow should the person not have adequate fat deposits at the donor site.

Anti-pollution skin products

I recently read in the newspaper that thirteen most polluted cities in the world are in India. This level of pollution, whether in the form of soot from vehicles, smog from industries or smoke from coal used to cook food in villages, cause a lot of damage to the skin. Blue light from computers, bacteria from heaters and air conditioners are other skin aggressors. There is a lot of research going on into the making of products which will protect the skin from pollution. Anti-pollution skincare range is going to sweep the markets.

Gel sheet masks

Dry sheet mask is applied to the face as is. It allows all the ingredients such as vitamins and hyaluronic acid to get absorbed into the skin and the mask is then removed after twenty minutes. These masks are easy to carry, easy to use and safe too. Gel sheet masks are used for an instant glow. Avoid if you have sensitive skin or a history of any allergy.

Charcoal masks

Charcoal masks contain bentonite clay and charcoal, which help in deep cleansing. These are good for people who have oily skin or pimple-prone skin or even combination skin. They reduce blackheads and whiteheads and also unclog pores. Charcoal masks make the skin dry, so people with dry or sensitive skin should not be using it.

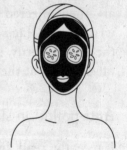

Charcoal mask

Glass skin

Glass skin, a term made popular by Korean beauties, is not a miracle. Glass skin is referred to crystal clear, blemish-free, translucent and radiant skin which looks like a piece of clear glass.

One cannot achieve glass skin overnight. It takes months of following a regular skincare regime to make your skin look like glass. But it is not impossible to achieve.

Steps to achieve glass skin—the K skincare

- At bedtime, remove all make-up from your face with a hydrating make-up remover or baby oil.
- Cleanse your face with a facewash that suits your skin type.
- Now apply a hydrating serum containing hyaluronic acid or vitamin C and vitamin E.
- Hydrating sheet masks (there are plenty of Korean brands to choose from) can also be used instead of serums.
- The serum or sheet mask is left overnight, allowing the skin to soak in the solution and enhancing complete absorption of the ingredients into the skin.
- In the morning, cleanse your face with plain water or a soap-free cleanser. Follow this with a moisturizer suitable for your skin type. Top it with a sunscreen which protects your skin from UVA and UVB rays.
- Make sure you avoid alcohol, nicotine and sugar.
- Sleep for at least six hours daily.
- Repeat this simple regime every single day for at least six months and you will see the transformation in your skin texture and tone.
- The results will be gratifying but the key is to maintain it by following these steps routinely.

The J skincare

Most people call me Dr J, so J skincare sounds like my skincare but it's not. It stands for Japanese skincare regime. J skincare is said to overpower the K (Korean) skincare by the end of 2018. The classic principles of Japanese aesthetics, kanso, shibui and seijaku—simplicity, understated beauty and *energetic* calm—take a natural course of skincare. Japanese skincare products, unlike the razzmatazz of Korean products, basically cater to everyday prevention. According to the Japanese, K beauty is more about trends and quick-fixes, while J beauty is more about technology-driven, holistic, traditional, preventive treatments. Time will tell us which is more powerful. Whatever it is, the basic skincare regime will not change.

Very often, my patients read about the latest treatments either on the Internet or in magazines, or hear it from friends and colleagues. Most of the time, however, these are not new treatments. They are simply old recipes in a new jar. Sometimes they are not even clinically proven treatments but are over-hyped and advertised. 'Doctor, my friend does Venus viva for her face, do you have it in your clinic?' my patient Rachel asked me once. Well, I have Endymed and Secret, both of which are devices using the same technology as Venus viva. Just as there are many cars in the market, from a Tata Nano to a Lamborghini, there are many lasers, radio frequency machines, HIFU devices and fat-freezing machines. While the underlying technology is the same, the make is different, hence the different names. So don't always check out what's new, check out what works. Before you follow the tribe and spend your hard-earned money on treatments that may not be necessary for you at all, do some research. Consult your dermatologist and let them decide what's best for you.

'Thank God for this lesson, now I won't get influenced by what people around me are doing to their skin. I'll just come and you do what's best for me. But don't forget to incorporate the newer technologies,' Mickey said at the end with a wink and a naughty smile on her face.

Epilogue

The Way Forward

'Genius is eternal patience'
—Michelangelo

Happiness speaks through the eyes and the skin too. Mickey looked like a fairy descended from heaven on her D-day. Her eyes emitted graciousness, her lips oozed charm, her beautiful skin seemed like it was radiating powerful positive energy from within and the joy on her face made her look ethereal. When I went up to wish her, she gave me the tightest hug and whispered, 'Thank you, Dr J. You are my angel.' Mickey had followed my advice and done all the treatments I had asked her to do like an obedient child.

Two months after her wedding, I saw her name in my appointment list. Had she spoilt her skin by eating all the wrong things or basking in the sun without sunscreen during her honeymoon, I wondered. But when she walked into my chamber, she looked as radiant and gorgeous as ever, with not a speck on her skin. She had even carried

all the supplements—sunscreen, moisturizer—to her
honeymoon as I had asked her to do. 'Doc, I came to
ask you if I needed to continue my skin routine. My skin
never looked so good and I didn't even tan as much on
my holiday,' she said. 'Mickey, you are a good child.
Yes, of course you need to follow your routine. Skin is
lifetime maintenance. Pollution, sunlight, stress and other
aggressors aren't going anywhere. They are right here to
spoil your skin if you don't take care.'

I gave Mickey a list of products to be used in summer
and another list in winter. 'Always remember, your skin
requirement changes according to the climate you are in,'
I told her. We made a checklist; her must-use products
were:

- Cleanser
- Make-up remover
- Moisturizer
- Sunscreen
- Vitamin C serum
- Under-eye cream
- Body lotion

We revised the skincare drill she had to embrace—from
healthy food, good sleep and exercise to meditation
and yoga. 'Doc, I do eat a lot of fresh fruits and green
vegetables, drink more water and coconut water. I have
given up sugar and processed food. I can already see the
difference not just in my skin, my body feels lighter too. I
have begun brisk-walking for half an hour in the morning
but I sleep on Sundays. I also make sure I get my six

hours of sleep,' she said. Superb, now all you have to do is follow this discipline for the rest of your life.

'Mickey, you will have to steer away from all the skin aggressors. Remember, the repercussions are not worth the momentary thrill. I'll be honest, it isn't going to be all that simple. It takes a little more than slathering sunscreen or eating right. The modern-day dramas of late-night parties, stress and pollution have to be tackled too. Make it a rule to avoid alcohol, or drink occasionally and only if necessary. Do not overindulge in smoking or drinking. Weed is not a fashion statement, it kills you and your skin.' Mickey and I went on a head-on agreement.

These six weeks, my friends, were not just Mickey's journey. It's the journey each one of us who desires to look beautiful from within and on the outside should take. And please do not take care of yourself to look good to others. You must look good to yourself and exude confidence. I hope you will take baby steps and gradually seep into the adulthood of flawless, graceful skin. An ounce of prevention is worth a pound of cure. This dictum of life holds true for our skin too. It is never too late for anything. Just like it is never too late to begin a new venture, never too late to say sorry, never too late to tell someone you love her, it is never too late to begin taking care of your skin, even if you are a guy. You will be amazed at what just a six-week routine can do to your skin. I do believe that we must age gracefully. But ageing gracefully does not mean sun spots, sagging skin and a haggard face.

I love to quote Coco Chanel in this context. She said, 'Nature gives you the face you have at twenty; it is up to you to merit the face you have at fifty.'

Don't wait for the assaults of pollution, stress and ageing to leave their trail on the skin. You should make skincare part of your routine. Just as you brush every day, bathe every day, comb your hair every day, you must cleanse, moisturize and use a sunscreen every day too. If you are good to your skin, it will remain loyal to you. Don't make it a few days' wonder like the gym you joined and quit after shedding those few pounds. You don't need exotic treatments and expensive creams. Trust me, committed holistic skincare will make heads turn even when you are seventy. Let the beauty in your heart and the beauty of your skin amalgamate to create a new ethereal you.

My love and best wishes to all.

Acknowledgements

'People who uplift you are the best kind of people. You don't simply keep them. You have to treasure them'

—Dodinsky

I want to first and foremost thank Shri Amitabh Bachchan from the bottom of my heart for his golden words of appreciation for the book and for being my sole inspiration in life.

I am eternally grateful to all the wonderful friends who have non-hesitantly given testimonials for my book. It means a lot to me.

To Milee Aishwarya for reinstilling my faith that doctors can become authors too.

To my lovely editor Gurveen Chadha for being the empathetic cop who guided me patiently all along my tenure as the author. This book would not have been possible without you.

To all those at Penguin Random House India who poured their blood, sweat and tears into the making of *Skin Rules*.

To Pooja Mertia for being the amazing creator of the book cover.

To my patients for being my biggest inspiration. And for being patient with me whenever I told them it would take more than six weeks for their skin to recover.

To my friends for always standing up for me and being my genuine ringmasters.

To my husband for being my punching bag for every snag and for standing tall like my Tower of Pisa I can always lean on.

To my father-in-law, Pinky, Chetan, Archit and Piyali for being my supporters all along.

To my sister who took over as brigadier of the Skinfiniti army and wing commander in my kitchen at home. While I had no time for anything but patients and this book in the last four months, she left no stone unturned in making sure my new Skinfiniti clinic has the swag. I moved in yesterday like a freshly appointed consultant.

To my adorable babies, Aarav and Giana, who were my sources of periodic entertainment when I felt my brain going kaput.

To my brother Sai Karun and sis-in-law Mili for being the perfect broadcast technicians whenever I wanted to chat with Giana just to overcome my mental blocks while writing this book.

To my staff for building Skinfiniti cooperative association; they have made sure I remain oblivious of any hiccups occurring at the clinic.

A big, heartfelt thank you once again. I promise to treasure all of you for the rest of my life.

A Note on the Author

DR JAISHREE SHARAD is the author of *Skin Talks*. She is India's leading celebrity cosmetic dermatologist, who has been practising for nineteen years. She is the only Indian on the board of directors of the International Society of Dermatologic and Aesthetic Surgery. She is also the international mentor of the American Society of Dermatologic Surgery. Jaishree is the founder and medical director of Skinfiniti Aesthetic Skin and Laser Clinic in Mumbai.

She is also the editor-in-chief of a cosmetic dermatology textbook called *Aesthetic Dermatology: Current Perspectives*, published in August 2018. She has been the vice president of the Cosmetic Dermatology Society of India for eight years. She was one of the '50 Outstanding Women in Health Care' at the World Health Congress Annual Awards in Mumbai in 2017.